'Woven with her knowledge as a doctor, as well as her own experiences as a mother, Punam pours so much heart into every page. A must read.'

GIOVANNA FLETCHER

'Dr Punam Krishan is the GP every mum wishes she had. This book will make so many mums feel seen, understood and supported. A powerful, important read for every woman.'

KIMBERLEY WALSH

'I wish I'd had this book when I had my babies – it should be available on the NHS! Dr Punam holds your hand on the rollercoaster that is early motherhood and way beyond.'

SARA COX

'This book is a gift to mothers everywhere. Combining GP expertise with honest, lived experience, The Mother Load is the book every mother should have on her bedside table.'

KATE LAWLER

'A brilliantly informative, uplifting and empowering book. I genuinely could not put it down.'

HELEN SKELTON

'Honest, reassuring and grounded in science – Dr Punam combines clinical insight with lived experience to explain what so many mothers feel but rarely hear discussed.'

DR AMIR KHAN

DR PUNAM KRISHAN

The Mother Load

EVERY MOTHER'S GUIDE TO JUGGLING HEALTH, LIFE & HAPPINESS

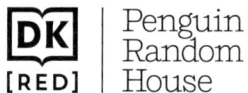

First published in Great Britain in 2026 by
DK RED, an imprint of
Dorling Kindersley Limited
20 Vauxhall Bridge Road,
London SW1V 2SA

The authorized representative in the EEA is
Dorling Kindersley Verlag GmbH. Arnulfstr. 124,
80636 Munich, Germany

A CIP catalogue record for this book
is available from the British Library.
ISBN: 978-0-2417-5638-6

Printed and bound in the United Kingdom

www.dk.com

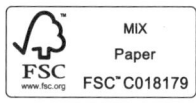

To Aarish and Ellora,

Thank you for everything you continue to teach me. Being your mum is the greatest honour of my life. I love you always.

And to every mother – you've got this x

Contents

Introduction

You might have picked up this book because you have just had a baby. The books, apps, online searches, and free-flowing advice that has come from everyone around you about your pregnancy and that first year have likely been helpful, but you are now curious about what happens next in your motherhood journey.

Perhaps you are feeling overwhelmed, exhausted, and lost in it all, and need some help to find yourself again. Maybe you are in the throes of motherhood and are seeking some guidance right now in what is a time of seismic change for you. Or it might be that you are many years down the line postnatally, but are still experiencing symptoms or complications from your birth. This might not even be about you at all – perhaps one of your mum friends, your daughter, or your sibling is impacted, or maybe you want to inform yourself for future birth experiences.

Whatever your reason for picking up this book, I want you to know that you are now my priority. This book is here to prepare you for any challenges that may lie ahead for you and your health, and to remind you to take care of yourself. Here's why.

My Story

Twelve years ago, I gave birth to my eldest child – my son, Aarish. After a healthy-ish pregnancy and, in my capacity as a doctor, feeling confident about what to expect, I went into labour. What happened next was an experience that turned our family's world upside down. I'll go into detail about what happened in Chapter 1, but, briefly, in 24 hours, I went from a healthy mum-to-be to being on a ventilator in intensive care with sepsis and multiple organ failure, my husband on the other side of a hospital with our newborn, feeling helpless and broken. My family were informed that I had days, perhaps hours, to live.

This was not how it was meant to be. No book I had read – as a doctor or in my prep for motherhood – had warned me about this. Miraculously, I pulled through, but not without scars – physical, mental, and emotional ones. However, what also came with that experience was a new-found appreciation for the word 'healing'.

For the first time in my career as a doctor, I found myself on the other side of the consultation table as a patient – a very vulnerable place to be. I was seeking answers, I needed support, and I was experiencing feelings that did not match up to what I had expected motherhood to be. I felt like I had failed at the one thing that was meant to come naturally to me, which left me wondering, 'What is wrong with me?' With a multitude of physical complications and on the edge with severe postnatal depression, I sat before my GP for my six-week postnatal check. I was in and out within a few minutes, all attention on the baby, and not even a consideration of how I was. Wow! When you already feel invisible, the one person who you need to notice you is your doctor. I realized there and then that there was a huge problem, and not just with my own consultation. As I chatted to other mums and heard how poor their postnatal care was, I knew I couldn't stay quiet.

This isn't me throwing shade at my GP, this is me – also a GP – acknowledging through lived experience what postnatal care actually looks like in many parts of the world. Across countries and health systems, the reality is stark: once the baby arrives, the spotlight often moves away from the mother entirely. Funding for maternal health services beyond birth is consistently under-prioritized. That's despite the fact that complications related to pregnancy and childbirth remain a leading cause of death and disability for women worldwide. When care stops at six weeks – or sometimes never even properly starts – we create the perfect conditions for the motherhood health penalty.

The Motherhood Health Penalty

It's no secret that gender bias in medicine has negatively impacted women for centuries. Historically, medical research and clinical trials have largely been conducted on male cells or using male volunteers, and so women have been underrepresented, which has led to gaps in our understanding of how diseases and medications affect them differently to men. Women have therefore received incorrect dosages of drugs which have only been trialled in men and they have been misdiagnosed due to a serious lack of education that signs and symptoms vary between men and women. Conditions like endometriosis, polycystic ovary syndrome (PCOS), adenomyosis, and menopause have been under researched, impacting women's fertility journeys and beyond.

There is even less education around maternal health. More than 40 million women every year experience health issues after giving birth which impact their health and well-being.[1] Sometimes, this could be for a few months, but, as a GP, I see these complications extend way beyond the postpartum phase. Often, women in their 40s and 50s admit to me that they have battled with incontinence or back pain, have not been intimate with their partners, or have struggled with their mood since the births of their children. When asked why they haven't come in sooner for help, they always say the same thing: 'I thought it was normal.'

This is the problem we have with the maternal health gap – due to inadequate awareness, research, and inclusion of mums in medical trials, due to the continued societal narrative of 'That's just what happens when you become a mum', due to the lack of teaching about the health of a mum postnatally during medical training, we have failed – and continue to fail – mothers. The mental load that comes with motherhood is often overlooked, dismissed, and attributed to anxiety, stress, or hysteria, rather than being thoroughly investigated for an underlying medical condition.

This is the motherhood health penalty and we need to speak about it and campaign for change. This book is my offering to this wider conversation.

About This Book

Most parenting or childcare books will take you to the year after childbirth, but, for many mums, at that time, healing has only just begun. What about their healthcare needs beyond this stage? What happens next?

Post-birth, a woman's body completely changes. She now has new aches and pains, and is battling fatigue on a level she has never known. Headaches, nausea, surgical scars, altered bowels, incontinence, painful sex, breast changes, and, of course, the peri/menopause are just some of the common complaints I hear about from my mum patients, and this does not include the mental load that nobody warns us about when we enter motherhood – and the invisible scars.

I spend a lot of time with female patients and one of my first screening questions is: 'Do you have any children?' This is such an important part of a medical consultation for me because, if the answer is yes, I already know that, no matter what stage of her motherhood journey she is at, her healthcare needs are different to everyone else's. Motherhood is a blessing; it is, however, also a risk factor for some medical problems. I don't want to be all doom and gloom because motherhood isn't that. Most of us will agree that becoming a mother is the best, most beautiful experience, but what I want to acknowledge is that it doesn't come without an impact on a woman's health and well-being.

There is a serious lack of information out there about maternal health through the decades and, in this book, I want to address that. Our health matters because if we mums stay well, our families stay well, we do our jobs well, and life goes well. It all starts, though, with us taking charge of us.

'Bouncing back' is a lie we've been sold. Motherhood is a lifelong journey that has a direct impact not just on your health, but on your relationships and interactions with the world around you that evolves over the years as you grow alongside your children. It's not just about adjusting to your 'new normal' because that normal is constantly changing and, as a GP, I want to be there for you, from both sides of the stethoscope and at every stage, because, as a mum, I know you often put yourself last.

Between those exhausted newborn nights and constantly evolving routines, it's easy to understand why new mums put their healthcare needs to one side – too busy, too tired, too worried it might be something, or too polite – not wanting to 'waste our time'. Most women think this phase will pass; however, what I have found is that the demands and to-do lists only get longer as the kids grow up – it is in the school-age era that I see most mums struggling to make time for themselves and their bodies, taking note only when things go wrong.

If that's you, this is your gentle reminder: you're never wasting our time. Your health matters just as much as everyone else's. You're allowed to get things checked. You deserve to feel well – not just push through. You deserve to make your health a priority now to prevent issues further down the line.

This book will help you do exactly that without adding to your to-do list. And just to say, when I use the word 'mum' throughout these pages, I mean *every* mum – whether you got here through birth, adoption, surrogacy, or foster care. This journey is yours, and your health matters.

One thing I always hear from my mum patients when it comes to maternal health goals is, 'I don't have time', but, hopefully, through this book, you will finally feel that you do. I have structured the chapters so you can dip in and out, focusing on the issues that you feel are most relevant to you right now, whether you're in the raw, teary newborn stage or the hormonal upheavals of peri/menopause (the Check-in that follows will help you to identify the areas to focus on).

We'll walk together through the decades of motherhood, looking at both the physical effects of becoming a mother, as well as how our mental health shifts along the way. We'll explore the changes that happen beneath the surface – from hormones and metabolism to muscles, joints, gut health, skin, sleep, and energy levels – along with the creeping anxiety, guilt, identity shifts, and deep-down fear that maybe you're not cut out for this after all. Most importantly, I'll be giving you the knowledge and tools to start supporting your body properly again, without guilt, pressure, or unrealistic expectations.

In each chapter, I've included a little bit of background to the common issues so many of my female patients come to me with, before diving into individual symptoms with quick hacks, tips, and habits that can help you to make simple changes one step at a time. I've also included a 'prescription' at the end of each chapter that outlines some simple changes you can weave into your day to positively impact your physical and emotional health. There are also patient examples and anecdotes throughout, as well as my personal story, so you can see how the micro changes I propose can really lead to major differences in the long term.

Motherhood is supposed to be instinctive, natural, and deeply fulfilling – at least that's the story we're often told. The truth is more complicated. From your first contraction to your little one's first day at school, from teenage mood swings to your own peri/

menopausal shifts, motherhood will test you in ways no antenatal class can prepare you for.

It changes you – your body, your mind, your priorities, your relationships. It can be exhilarating and beautiful. It can also be overwhelming, frightening, and exhausting. Some days, you'll feel capable and calm. Other days, you'll wonder if you're falling apart.

I am a mum of two and I really do get it. It's time to prioritize your health alongside your family's so you can all thrive together.

The Check-in

It can be hard to know what's normal and what's not when it comes to physical and mental health. Crikey, I'm a doctor and even I don't always know!

Something I have found over the last 20 years as a doctor, though, is that mums accept many symptoms as being normal. Because we have little understanding of what actually happens to us beyond pregnancy and childbirth, we can assume that everything that follows is just to be expected. The issue is that generations above us have also not been told and so stories get passed along, mums talk in groups, and, within those echo chambers, everything – including the abnormal symptoms – becomes normalized.

I love a checklist and, below, I've included some important questions to ask yourself to help identify any issues that might be lingering post-birth – months, or even years, down the line. This will enable you to gauge your baseline and know which chapters to focus on first. I also hope it will give you an easy toolkit to help you have a conversation about the way you are feeling with your doctor or other healthcare professional.

When answering these questions, please try to be honest – it's great if you're feeling great, but, if you are not, that's OK too. Many mums find things hard, so open up. The longer you struggle in silence, the harder things will feel.

While doing your 'Mama MOT', have a think about your family history. Some conditions can often be triggered by or during pregnancy, and so sharing your family history with your doctor can be helpful should any new symptoms appear. Examples include diabetes, heart disease, autoimmune conditions, neurological conditions, or cancer.

Your Physical Health

- ❏ Do you feel you haven't fully recovered from childbirth? *(Chapter 3)*
- ❏ Have any wounds or scars healed or are you worried about them? *(Chapter 3)*
- ❏ Do you suspect you have muscle separation in your abdomen (known as *diastasis recti*)? *(Chapter 5)*
- ❏ Are you tired all the time? *(Chapter 2)*
- ❏ Do you have trouble falling or staying asleep, or are you sleeping too much? *(Chapter 3)*
- ❏ Do you have any abnormal vaginal discharge? *(Chapter 3)*
- ❏ Do you have any concerns about your current bleeding pattern? *(Chapter 3)*
- ❏ Are you managing to go to the toilet? Do you have any problems passing urine/opening your bowels? *(Chapter 3)*
- ❏ Have you had sex since your baby was born? Do you have any physical concerns around this? *(Chapter 4)*
- ❏ Have your breasts changed since giving birth? *(Chapter 3)*
- ❏ Do you have any skin concerns? *(Chapter 10)*
- ❏ Did you have any joint issues when you were pregnant and are they still lingering? *(Chapter 5)*

Your Mental Health

- ❑ Do you feel nervous, anxious, or on edge? *(Chapter 7)*
- ❑ Are you crying all the time? *(Chapter 7)*
- ❑ Do you feel down, depressed, or hopeless? *(Chapter 7)*
- ❑ Have you had any negative thoughts about you or your baby? *(Chapter 7)*
- ❑ Was your birth traumatic? *(Chapter 1)*
- ❑ Are you having any flashbacks from your birth? *(Chapter 1)*
- ❑ Do you feel you haven't bonded with your baby? *(Chapter 1)*
- ❑ Do you feel worried all the time? *(Chapter 8)*
- ❑ Do you have any concerns about your memory or difficulty concentrating? *(Chapter 6)*
- ❑ Do you feel continually stressed? *(Chapter 8)*
- ❑ Do you feel overwhelmed? *(Chapter 8)*
- ❑ Are you feeling strong negative emotions such as fear, anger, failure, guilt, or shame? *(Chapter 7)*
- ❑ Do you feel isolated or distant from other people? *(Chapter 9)*
- ❑ Are there any challenges in your relationship with your partner and/or family and friends? *(Chapter 8)*

It's important to note that if you develop any new symptoms or have ongoing concerns, please don't be tempted to ask Dr Google and self-diagnose, ignore them, or assume they'll get better in time. Let your doctor know and they will assess whether it's important or not and, at the very least, it's always good to have any health concerns recorded in your notes.

I know that going to the doctor can sometimes be quite overwhelming and can even be stressful because you worry about all the 'what ifs': *What if they think I'm stupid? What if they judge me? What if I'm wasting their time?*

I promise you we think none of these things. However, if you don't raise your concerns, your doctor will never know and you might risk suffering in silence, which won't help you or your family in the long term. Please ask all the questions – nothing is ever silly.

'I Had a Difficult Birth'

HEALING FROM BIRTH TRAUMA

The story we tell about birth is often incomplete. I learnt this when I became a mother myself. We talk about contractions, the big moment of delivery, the weight of the baby, and the cuddles. We post the pictures, recount the funny bits, and tend to gloss over the rest. While this is a reality for many, sadly, for a huge number of women, birth doesn't feel magical. It feels terrifying. Disorienting. Traumatic. Disconnected. And deeply lonely.

While I understand that not every mother's journey begins with trauma, mine did – and it shaped everything that followed. That's why I've chosen to open this book with the moment everything changes: the moment you meet your baby, the moment a new version of you is born, and the moment the mother load begins.

Even if your birth was calm or straightforward, I hope you'll see that this chapter covers more than trauma – it speaks to the identity shift, the emotional intensity, and the physical and mental rupture that birth can bring, in big or small ways. This is where the journey starts for so many women: with a body that's just been through something enormous, a mind that's trying to make sense of it, and a heart that's suddenly carrying more than it ever has before. So, even if the details differ, the deeper truth unites us: becoming a mother is a profound shift. And it deserves to be acknowledged, honestly, from the very beginning.

The Different Types of Maternal Scars

Globally, up to 45 per cent of new mothers have experienced a traumatic birth.[1] In the UK, one in three women describe the birth of their child as traumatic[2] and around 30,000 women each year meet full diagnostic criteria for post-traumatic stress disorder (PTSD) after giving birth[3]. And these are only the cases we *know* about; I suspect the actual numbers are higher.

Birth trauma can be physical, psychological, or both. It is often an entanglement of fear, pain, loss of control, shame, and inadequately supported medical interventions. It can be as acute as a life-threatening haemorrhage or as quiet as a woman feeling unheard during labour. It can happen in a long, dramatic emergency or during what is documented as a 'normal birth'.

Birth also leaves behind more than one kind of scar. There are the visible scars from the caesarean incision, the episiotomy wound, the stitches, or the swelling. Then there are deep physical injuries such as pelvic floor trauma, tears, nerve damage, prolapse, anal sphincter injuries, or bladder dysfunction, all of which we'll look at in the chapters to come.

But deeper still, there are the invisible scars – the ones no one sees. The ones hidden inside the nervous system. The ones that come out at night in the form of flashbacks and panic. The ones that whisper 'You failed' even when you didn't. The ones that shake your confidence as a mother, a partner, or a woman. These invisible wounds can shape a mother's experience for years, often influencing her physical health, emotional wellbeing, self-confidence, relationships, and even how she experiences hormonal shifts like peri/menopause decades later.

My own story: A doctor on the other side of the table

As a GP, I thought I understood difficult births. I'd seen tears, emergencies, and complex deliveries. I'd held women's hands while they cried through their postnatal checks. I knew the clinical language, the guidelines, and the risks.

Then I had my son.

My pregnancy had been relatively OK. I was previously fit and well, and there were no anticipated issues from my prenatal team. On the day of delivery, I ended up with a very long and complicated labour. A series of missed opportunities, delays, and poor communication led to an emergency forceps delivery. I sustained a 3B tear, which, as we'll see in Chapter 3, is a severe obstetric anal sphincter injury and affects the muscles that control continence. At the same time, I became critically unwell, with a life-threatening haemorrhage, a blood transfusion reaction causing anaphylaxis, followed by sepsis and multiple organ failure. I went from the anticipation and excitement of meeting my precious baby to hearing the words, 'We are losing her' from the anaesthetist, and multiple doctors and theatre nurses trying to resuscitate me. I spent a week in intensive care and woke up a changed person.

Clinically, the team acted fast to save my life. The medical focus was, of course, survival, but, emotionally, a lot of damage took place. I felt broken by my birth. This was not how I had imagined I would be welcoming my beautiful son into the world.

When I woke up, I was told about the repair to control the bleeding 'down below'. I was attached to a million tubes and machines beeping away, my body all swollen and my baby nowhere to be seen. That was the moment that broke me.

I looked at my husband, helpless. I didn't recognize myself. I didn't recognize my body. I didn't feel like a mother; I felt like a patient clinging to life while everyone around me looked on in pity. While everyone celebrated the birth of my son, a truly joyous moment, the reality was that this birth had nearly killed me.

There was just too much to process. Too much shock and grief and guilt, but the strongest emotion was shame – a shame I couldn't logically justify, but that I deeply felt. A shame that whispered: 'Your body failed the one thing it was meant to do. *You* failed.'

It took a long time and A LOT of help and support to find myself and my health again, but one thing I learnt along the way was that it was not my fault.

A birth trauma experience is never your fault. It is a hugely unfair and unfortunate experience, but it is nothing that you did or failed at.

Being a doctor on the other side of the table added another layer to the trauma I felt. I knew the risks of such tears. I knew what chronic pelvic floor injury could mean. I knew the postpartum complications of sepsis. I knew the statistics. My medical brain bombarded me with catastrophic 'what ifs', but I also saw, first-hand, how limited postnatal support actually was. I saw the huge gaps in a way I had never seen before, and I could not unsee them.

The gaps in our system

Despite advances in maternity care, several painful gaps still persist today. In the UK alone, we are faced with:

1. **Communication failure:** One of the strongest predictors of birth trauma is poor communication – being moved between staff, not having procedures explained, and feeling dismissed or unheard.
2. **Postnatal care is too limited:** A single six-week check cannot possibly address:
   - pelvic floor function
   - sexual health
   - continence concerns
   - emotional well-being
   - birth trauma
   - breastfeeding struggles
   - hormonal shifts
   - wound healing
     Most women leave that appointment with unanswered questions.

3. **Birth trauma is minimized:** Women are told: 'At least the baby is healthy', 'All births are hard', 'This is normal' – statements that are meant to reassure, but often silence trauma instead.

4. **Pelvic injuries are underdiagnosed:** Evidence suggests that a significant proportion of obstetric anal sphincter injuries (severe perineal tears) are not recognized at the time of delivery. In one study, clinical examination and imaging after birth increased detection of these injuries from approximately 11 per cent to 24.5 per cent, indicating many tears were initially missed at routine assessment.[4] Missed injuries cause years of complications.

5. **Mental health support is limited:** Many women experiencing birth trauma or PTSD are misdiagnosed with generalized anxiety or depression, or not diagnosed at all. Over 40 per cent of mothers in the UK felt that their GP did not spend enough time talking to them about their mental health.[5]

6. **Trauma echoes across decades:** Women often re-experience symptoms in:
   - perimenopause (due to hormonal changes affecting pelvic tissue)
   - menopause (vaginal dryness, changes in continence, pain)
   - future pregnancies
   - smear tests (see page 30 for support with that first smear after birth)
   - sexual intimacy
   - medical examinations

Trauma doesn't follow the NHS six-week healing timeline. It follows its own and requires those around you to pick up the signs.

The lifelong ramifications of birth trauma

Birth trauma doesn't just affect the early postpartum days, it shapes a woman's health across her entire life.

Physical impacts
- pelvic floor dysfunction
- anal incontinence
- chronic pelvic pain
- painful sex
- prolapse
- bladder urgency or leakage
- bowel issues
- nerve damage
- hormonal sensitivities later in life

Mental health impacts
- postnatal PTSD
- hypervigilance
- panic attacks
- low mood or postnatal depression
- flashbacks
- nightmares
- perinatal anxiety
- avoidance of medical settings
- birth-related phobias (such as tokophobia – a severe fear of birth)

These symptoms often overlap with sleep deprivation, making recovery even harder.

Sexual health impacts
- pain during sex

- fear
- flashbacks
- body image concerns
- loss of libido
- trauma linked to touch

All of these are incredibly common yet rarely discussed and carry much stigma.

Relationship impacts

- partners don't know how to help and communication breaks down
- mothers withdraw emotionally because they're overwhelmed, ashamed, or still in shock
- birth partners experience trauma too, but often feel they cannot share it

Future reproductive decisions

- women choose not to have more children because they fear another birth, they fear complications again, or they have a very real fear of dying
- many women simply cannot imagine going through it again emotionally

Medical avoidance

This is HUGE! Women who have experienced birth trauma frequently avoid:

- doctor's appointments
- smear tests
- postnatal checks
- pelvic exams
- contraception reviews

- physiotherapy
- sexual health care

Avoiding medical care leads to worse long-term outcomes, compounding trauma further. It also puts women at risk of missing serious conditions by avoiding screening appointments.

Before we go any further, it is important I say this: trauma does not and must not ever compare. Your story does not have to be as 'bad' as someone else's to count. No one else gets to minimize your pain. Trauma is not defined by clinical notes. It is defined by the emotional experience.

There is NO hierarchy of birth trauma. There is no 'too little' and no 'too big'. No one else has the right to decide whether your birth was traumatic – only YOU do.

If your birth frightened you, overwhelmed you, or left you feeling powerless, unheard, or violated, it was trauma – and I have written this chapter for you. Your experience is valid. Your healing matters and you are not alone.

'I Don't Understand What Happened and Feel Like a Failure'

One of the most common things women tell me in clinic after a difficult birth is some version of, 'I don't really know what happened.' The memories feel jumbled, the sequence feels out of order, and things often feel blurred. They remember the fear, the urgency, and the pain, but not the explanations. They remember the faces leaning over them, but not the words. They recall smells of the environment, but can't quite locate where they were. They remember making decisions without understanding what they were agreeing to. They remember the panic in the room, the lights, the beeps, and the silence afterwards.

When you don't understand what happened, your mind tries to make sense of the trauma and fills in the blanks, often with self-blame:

- 'My body didn't work.'
- 'I couldn't do what other women can.'
- 'I wasn't strong enough.'
- 'I should have known what to do.'
- 'I should have pushed better.'
- 'I let everyone down.'

This is what we have been taught by society, but the truth is that birth is not a test and you cannot fail it. Birth is a complex physiological process. No amount of positive thinking, yoga breathing, or planning can control the position of the baby, the length of the labour, the timing of contractions, the placenta, the cord, your pelvis, or the progress of an emergency. Your body is not a machine. It can't follow a script, although, sometimes, some books, or indeed antenatal groups and classes, might have you believe there is one.

Women so often blame themselves because society romanticizes birth as something that should be instinctive and natural – an empowering ceremony where your body just 'knows exactly what to do'. So, naturally, when things go off-course, you assume it's all your fault when it isn't. Birth is unpredictable. Complications are common. Interventions save lives. Feeling like a failure is a symptom of trauma, not a reflection of reality.

So many women misunderstand their own birth – for various reasons:

- **Pain affects memory:** During intense pain, the brain prioritizes survival. It does not record memories clearly and many mothers only retain fragments of what happened during labour and birth.

- **Fear distorts perception:** Fear heightens the amygdala (the brain's alarm centre). When the alarm is going off, the reasoning part of the brain switches off and so you might not be able to process information properly.
- **Communication in labour is inconsistent:** With staff changes, shift swaps, and emergencies escalating, it's all going on! Sometimes explanations are rushed or missed, and sometimes no one explains what's happening at all. Research shows that poor communication is one of the strongest predictors of birth trauma.[6]
- **You lose your sense of agency:** When interventions pile up quickly – induction, drip, monitoring, epidural, ventouse, forceps, episiotomy, caesarean section (C-section) – it can feel like things are happening *to* you, not *with* you. Loss of control is profoundly traumatic.
- **Dissociation:** Many women mentally detach during a traumatic birth. You might physically be there but feel 'outside your body', watching it happen from afar. Dissociation protects you but leaves huge memory gaps.
- **You were prioritizing survival:** For some women, especially after emergency C-sections, postpartum haemorrhage (PPH), or foetal distress, the focus becomes 'just get us through this', and so it is difficult to store a coherent narrative while fighting for safety.

On top of all this, the silence afterwards makes everything worse. After a traumatic birth, you often don't get the time or space to process it. You're whisked into newborn care, breastfeeding challenges, sleep deprivation, visitors, check-ups, nappies, and feeding schedules. Meanwhile, you have just gone through a life-altering event that your brain cannot even fully comprehend yet.

Rarely does anyone sit you down to explain the medical details or talk you through what the midwives or doctors saw. While everyone means well, they get caught up in the joy of the new baby, assume you are well, and don't check-in on how you are emotionally. It is heartbreaking how many women spend years believing they 'failed' when they simply didn't get an explanation. I am one of them.

I have met women in my clinic in their 40s and 50s who still cry when describing births that happened decades ago because they were never told what actually happened. They carried shame instead of understanding. It doesn't have to be this way.

What you can do

- **Speak to someone:** You were not meant to hold this silently. Talking is powerful. Trauma processed aloud becomes less threatening to the brain. You can speak to:
  - a trusted friend
  - your partner
  - your family doctor
  - your health visitor
  - a therapist
  - a postnatal support group
  - another mum who understands

  You don't have to narrate the whole story at once, but even naming one part of the experience can begin to heal the pain. Speak the truth of what happened. Trauma shrinks in the light.
- **Write down everything you remember:** Not beautifully. Not neatly. Just write it.
  - 'What I remember …'
  - 'What I felt …'
  - 'What no one explained …'
  - 'What I still don't understand …'

  Writing helps your brain join the dots and stops the thoughts and memories from looping.

- **Ask for your maternity notes:** The law differs across the world, but, at the time of writing, in the UK, Europe, and the US, you are legally entitled to your health records. Your maternity notes will help to:
  - fill in gaps
  - explain interventions
  - clarify decisions
  - give context
  - help you understand the clinical side

  So many women feel immediate relief once they see that they did nothing wrong.
- **Consider trauma-focused therapy:** Birth trauma is trauma and it responds beautifully to early therapeutic support such as:
  - trauma-focused cognitive behavioural therapy (TF-CBT)
  - eye movement desensitization and reprocessing (EMDR)
  - trauma-informed counselling

  These therapies help your brain to file the memory properly, reducing flashbacks, panic, guilt, and shame. Therapy rewires the fear centres of the brain and helps you rebuild safety.

'My Birth Broke Me'

When a woman says, 'My birth broke me', she isn't being dramatic. She is telling the emotional truth of a moment that reshaped her physically and psychologically. Birth trauma can look like:

- flashbacks
- nightmares
- panic attacks
- intrusive images
- feelings of dread
- fear of going to sleep

- fear of your baby crying
- difficulty bonding
- numbness
- rage
- loss of pleasure
- feeling disconnected from your body
- avoiding sex
- avoiding smear tests
- avoiding hospitals
- avoiding future pregnancies

You can be a loving mother *and* still feel broken by your birth. Yes, those two experiences can exist side by side.

When you've had a traumatic birth, it can feel like your sense of self fractures. Mothers often describe it to me in clinic as:

- 'I feel like something inside me cracked.'
- 'I don't feel like myself.'
- 'I left part of me in that delivery room.'
- 'I feel broken in a way no one can see.'

I totally get it. That's the thing about birth trauma, it is often invisible. No one sees the emotional wounds when you're holding a newborn. No one sees the terror that rises when someone says 'forceps'. No one sees you freeze when you pass the hospital. No one sees the ache in your chest when you try to talk about what happened or hear how other women 'sailed through it'. You look 'fine' from the outside, but, inside, you are trying to rebuild yourself from the pieces.

The emotional reality of birth trauma

Birth trauma fractures a woman's psychological foundation in three main ways:

1. **Lack of safety:** Your sense of physical safety is shaken:
   - Your body did things you didn't expect.
   - Pain overwhelmed you.
   - Medical emergencies happened.
   - You felt out of control.
2. **Loss of identity:** Women tell me: 'I don't know who I am anymore.' Birth trauma can disconnect you from the confident, capable woman you were before. Your sense of identity feels replaced by fear, exhaustion, and uncertainty.
3. **Loss of trust:** Many women feel they have lost trust – in their body, in their instincts, in their care providers, and in the process. Sometimes, they have even lost trust in their own emotions.

I want you to remember: you didn't become fragile; something frightening happened to you. BUT, you are still strong. You are still whole. You are still you. You just need healing.

What the science says

Birth trauma is a legitimate neurophysiological response to overwhelming distress. When a woman feels endangered in labour – whether physically or emotionally – the amygdala goes into overdrive, the stress hormone cortisol floods the system, and the rational part of the brain (the prefrontal cortex) shuts down. You go into survival mode. This is why trauma symptoms often resemble those seen after car accidents, assaults, or medical emergencies.

After birth, especially traumatic birth, your system remains on high alert. You may experience:

- feeling constantly on edge
- jumpiness

- difficulty sleeping
- racing thoughts
- emotional numbness
- hypervigilance ('danger is everywhere')
- panic or dread
- tearfulness

This is your nervous system trying to protect you, but doing so in overdrive.

Birth trauma isn't just emotional – many women also deal with untreated or under-treated physical complications that compound the emotional load. The most common ones I see as a GP are:

- perineal tears and pelvic floor injuries (see page 96)
- bladder trauma and birth-related incontinence (see page 73)
- prolapse (see page 79)
- chronic pain: pain can persist due to scar tissue (see page 96), nerve injury, muscle imbalance, vaginal dryness (see page 101), pelvic floor tension (see page 96), or unresolved trauma stored in the body
- C-section complications (see page 70)
- postpartum haemorrhage and severe complications: women who experience major haemorrhage, sepsis, emergency surgery, or ICU admission often deal with flashbacks, panic, avoidance of hospitals, survivor's guilt, and fear of future pregnancies. Your 'clinical emergency' has emotional consequences.

Why traumatic birth affects bonding

Bonding with your baby doesn't always come instantly, especially when your body and mind are recovering from trauma. Women often carry guilt for this, thinking:

- 'I didn't feel that rush of love! What's wrong with me?'
- 'I felt nothing at first – am I broken?'

Nothing is wrong with you. Your brain was trying to survive. Love arrives in many ways, often slowly and quietly, and that's OK. You and your baby will find your way because bonding doesn't require a perfect birth, it requires time, safety, and connection; all things you can rebuild.

How birth trauma affects the body through the decades

Something important to note is that birth trauma does not 'expire'. It evolves.

In your 20s and early motherhood, it can lead to:

- pain
- incontinence
- pelvic heaviness
- low confidence
- fear of sex
- fear of another birth

In your 30s:

- considering more children becomes emotionally complex
- anxiety resurfaces
- heavier periods can worsen prolapse symptoms

In your 40s (perimenopause), you might notice that:

- hormonal changes unmask old pelvic injuries
- vaginal dryness increases pain
- urgency or leakage worsens
- libido changes feel emotionally charged
- old trauma triggers more easily

In your 50s and beyond (menopause and post-menopause):

- scar tissue becomes more rigid and painful due to thinning vaginal walls, making sex or even smear tests more uncomfortable
- nerve sensitivity from old perineal injuries can be amplified by hormonal changes
- prolapse symptoms (such as a bulging feeling or pelvic heaviness – see page 79) may worsen as the connective tissues lose support
- urinary incontinence may become more frequent or severe
- emotional trauma can resurface unexpectedly

Women frequently think these symptoms are 'just menopause', but it is often menopause layered over childbirth injury. As oestrogen levels decline, the tissues of the vulva, vagina, and pelvic floor become thinner, drier, and less elastic. This is called genitourinary syndrome of menopause (GSM), and it's incredibly common but still not talked about enough. If you've experienced a birth injury, such as a tear, episiotomy, pelvic floor trauma, or forceps delivery, those areas of your body may already have scar tissue, nerve sensitivity, or structural weakness. When menopause arrives and oestrogen levels drop, these previously injured areas often become more symptomatic.

This is why it is vital that women are given support to process birth trauma, whatever decade they are in.

What you can do

- **Plan future births with trauma-informed care:** If you
  choose another pregnancy:
  - ○ ask for consultant-led care
  - ○ request continuity of midwife
  - ○ plan a gentle C-section if preferred
  - ○ ask for trauma-informed support
  - ○ do not be afraid to say what you need

  You are allowed to protect yourself.
- **Strengthen your support network:** Connection heals
  trauma. Isolation worsens it. Reach out. (See Chapter 9 for
  more on the importance of connection.)
- **Consider hormonal support:** This is particularly relevant
  in perimenopause. Oestrogen (if there are no specific
  reasons for you not to take it, known as
  'contraindiciations') can help with:
  - ○ vaginal dryness
  - ○ pain
  - ○ bladder symptoms
  - ○ tissue health

The dreaded smear

After you've had your baby, it's a good time to check if your
smear is up to date, especially if you have missed it due to
pregnancy. Sadly, something I hear from women who have
experienced traumatic births is that they haven't been able
to attend their routine smears in years, they fear internal
examinations, and, even more painfully, hold back on their
dreams to have more children.

If you have been through a difficult birth, live with pelvic
pain, incontinence, or vaginismus (more on these in later
chapters), then speculums and exams can feel unbearable.

You are not weak or failing – this is your body subconsciously trying to protect you from any more pain.

There is help and support to treat this, but you need to reach out and speak to your doctor. I know this not just as a GP, but as a woman who went through it myself after the birth of my first child. I'd had a difficult delivery, and although my body had healed on the outside, the thought of anything invasive – even a routine smear test – filled me with dread. I avoided it for a long time. I was scared it would hurt, that it would trigger flashbacks, or that I'd feel out of control again. And, for a while, I told myself it could wait. But, eventually, I asked for help. I got the support I needed, I had counselling, and I slowly began to rebuild that trust in my body. I still get a bit nervous and uptight before a smear test, so I ask my GP for a low-dose muscle relaxant like diazepam – and that's OK. Breathing exercises help immensely during the test, and I always leave feeling reassured in my body. I went on to have another baby, and I no longer avoid essential screening. These tests are vital and life-saving. I don't want any woman putting herself at risk because of fear, pain, or past trauma – especially when compassionate, trauma-informed care is available.

Aside from counselling, there are some things you can do to help make that first smear after birth a little easier, such as creating a calming playlist, taking someone with you for support, or doing breathing exercises to help you relax. It's also so important to be open and honest with the team carrying out the smear so they're in the know and can help put you at ease throughout.

Punam's Prescription

Ask for a birth debrief

Many hospitals offer a birth afterthoughts or birth reflections service. You can request this and sit with a midwife or obstetrician who will:

- go through your notes with you
- explain the timeline
- answer your questions
- help you interpret what happened
- clarify that nothing was 'your fault'

A birth debrief helps your brain process trauma and reduces guilt. It is an emotional and clinical reset – a chance to say, 'This is my story, and I deserve to understand it.' We know that debriefing can help improve mental health outcomes postnatally. If your hospital doesn't offer it, your doctor can help you request your notes and support you to make sense of them.

These appointments can be emotional, so it's a good idea to take someone with you. Having someone beside you helps with:

- absorbing information
- emotional grounding
- asking questions you might forget
- making you feel safe

Knowledge is grounding. Understanding is healing.

Hold space for yourself

You survived something massive – physically, emotionally, and psychologically. Whether your birth was textbook or traumatic, it marked a profound shift in your life. The exhaustion, the tears, and the vivid memories, or numbness are not signs of weakness. They're signs of survival. Your feelings are valid. You are allowed to grieve parts of your birth, even if others say, 'At least the baby's OK.'

Ask for help early

If something doesn't feel right – physically or mentally – please don't wait. Therapy, pelvic health physiotherapy, trauma-informed care, and birth reflections services are all tools, not signs of failure. The sooner you ask, the sooner healing can begin. There's no medal for doing it all alone, but there is relief in being supported.

Final Thoughts

Know this: you are not broken.

You are healing. You are rising. You are becoming someone stronger than the woman who walked into that birth room.

And you truly deserve to – and can – feel whole again.

CHAPTER 2

'I'm Tired All the Time'

COPING WITH EXHAUSTION

'I am knackered! Shattered! Exhausted! Broken! So tired!'

I am a mum to two kids, a twelve-year-old and a five-year-old, at the time of writing. The dog is a middle child and just as needy, so I shall add him to the list. Maybe the husband too? OK, so I have four dependents ... and here is how my everyday goes:

I call my mum on the way to school drop-off and tell her how tired I am. She is 61, and she tells me how tired she is too – we moan about it and wish each other a good day. On the way to work, I call my best friend who is also a mum. We tell each other how exhausted we are, moan about all the millions of things we have to do and haven't done, and wish each other a good day. We say 'the juggle is real' at least once a day. I feel validated, and sometimes that by itself can help – I know I am not alone. I then get into clinic and I cannot tell you how many mothers share their fatigue burdens with me. This includes my staff as well as my patients. While we all lead different lives and have diverse experiences and circumstances, the common thread is the exhaustion that comes from navigating mum life.

One thing I have observed in all my interactions and experiences is how the anatomy and physiology of tiredness changes throughout the seasons of motherhood. Maternal fatigue is a phenomenon that affects many women during pregnancy, the postpartum phase, and beyond. In this chapter, I want to really get to the heart of that overwhelming, deep, and persistent exhaustion that affects a mother's physical, emotional, and mental well-being, and give you some practical tools to help ease it. This chapter is a biggie as tiredness is something that affects so many mums across the board.

Before we get stuck in, let's look at the science behind maternal fatigue and why it happens.

The Science of Maternal Fatigue

Maternal exhaustion is frequently overlooked because society has long normalized it as just being part of parenting, often gaslighting women if they ever complain about it, which has led to a lack of solutions and, more importantly, support – whether that's at home, in the community, or at work. Any mother going through it will describe it as a deep feeling that nothing seems to fix.

What I have learnt in my 20 years as a doctor is that maternal fatigue is more than just 'feeling tired' and it can manifest in various ways. There are the physical symptoms of persistent tiredness, such as daytime exhaustion, reduced energy levels, headaches, and aches and pains in joints. Then there are the cognitive impairments, including brain fog (which we'll explore in detail in Chapter 6 – see page 143), difficulty concentrating, and memory lapses. Lastly, there are the emotional effects of fatigue which include increased irritability, mood swings, anxiety, worry, feelings of overwhelm, and anger. In fact, there is even a condition known as 'depleted mother syndrome', which is when mums feel totally drained, both physically and emotionally, often leading to burnout.[1]

And the common causes of maternal fatigue are just as varied – I'm sure some of those described below will resonate with you!

Hormonal changes

Fluctuating hormones like progesterone can increase levels of sleepiness and fatigue during pregnancy, but this also occurs during your periods, which can change significantly after you have a baby. They may return to pre-pregnancy patterns but not always – for a number of reasons:

- **Changes to the hypothalamic–pituitary–ovarian (HPO) axis:** Pregnancy and postpartum can rewire the signalling pathway between your brain and ovaries. This can affect how regularly or strongly hormones are released. Oestrogen may remain lower if periods don't return regularly, for example, due to extended breastfeeding, stress, weight fluctuations, or approaching perimenopause.
- **Periods themselves might change:** After pregnancy, your uterine lining, cervix, and pelvic floor are all affected which can make periods heavier, lighter, more painful, or more irregular. These changes reflect shifts in hormone sensitivity and balance.
- **Age and perimenopause:** If you've had children in your 30s or early 40s, your body may already be in the early stages of perimenopause – a time when hormone levels (especially oestrogen and progesterone) start to fluctuate naturally. This means your post-baby hormones might already be on a new trajectory.

Furthermore, as you enter the peri/menopausal seasons, these fluctuations can make you feel slow, heavy, tired all the time, and drained of energy.

Tracking your cycle and, more importantly, the symptoms you have is vital to help you and your doctor determine whether the cause of your fatigue is hormonal (see box overleaf).

Cycle tracking

There are lots of free and accessible online apps and menstrual trackers you can use to track your cycle and symptoms. Alternatively, keep a paper journal, noting:

- **The first and last day of your period:** This helps determine your cycle length and whether it's regular. Short, long, or inconsistent cycles can flag hormone imbalances, thyroid issues, or early perimenopause.
- **The flow (spotting, light, moderate, heavy):** Changes in flow can signal shifts in hormone levels, fibroids, polyps, or the effects of contraception. Very heavy or very light periods are worth discussing with your doctor.
- **Mood (low, irritable, anxious, energized):** Hormones like oestrogen, progesterone, and serotonin fluctuate across your cycle – this impacts your mood. Patterns of premenstrual syndrome (PMS) or premenstrual dysphoric disorder (PMDD – severe mood changes before your period) can become clearer with tracking.
- **Sleep (quality, quantity, interruptions, hot flushes, and night sweats):** Sleep disturbances – especially in the second half of your cycle – can be linked to progesterone and oestrogen levels. Night sweats or insomnia may also point to perimenopause or thyroid issues.
- **Energy levels (high, average, low, exhausted):** Energy dips often follow hormonal changes – for example, progesterone rising after ovulation can cause fatigue. Persistent low energy could indicate low iron, B12, thyroid imbalance, or chronic stress.
- **Cognitive function (sharp, foggy, forgetful):** 'Brain fog' can correlate with hormone fluctuations, especially during the luteal phase, postpartum, or perimenopause. Tracking

helps doctors to connect cognitive symptoms with your cycle pattern.

- **Physical symptoms (bloating, cramps, headaches, joint pain, breast pain, urine infections, and so on):** These help us spot hormonal triggers, inflammatory patterns, or underlying conditions like endometriosis, fibroids, or fluctuating oestrogen. Breast pain, for instance, is common in the luteal phase.

And don't forget the in-between symptoms:

- **Mid-cycle spotting, vaginal discharge, and libido shifts:** These can help identify when (or if) you're ovulating, which is key for fertility, contraception, and cycle regulation.
- **Changes to cycle patterns:** Sudden irregularity, missed periods, or shorter/longer cycles can suggest perimenopause, stress, weight changes, thyroid, or other hormone-related conditions.

Bringing this kind of tracking to your doctor's appointment will give them a clear window into your hormonal health, which is much more valuable than a single blood test on one day of your cycle. It helps them to spot trends, patterns, and possible diagnoses much faster.

Physical demands

The body's continuous adjustments – whether that is to growing a baby, repairing and healing after birth, or in the years beyond as complications such as pelvic/back pain, prolapses, or incontinence may have developed – all take their toll on a woman's body. The sleepless nights which span years – whether that is due to lack of sleep or worry and stress – also drain our energy and contribute to background inflammation.

Inflammation is the body's natural response to dealing with any form of stress, injury, trauma, or infection. Its job is to protect the body and help heal the area that is affected. In the short term, inflammation is not a serious issue; however, if left unmanaged over a long period of time, it can quietly wear us down, which can happen in exhausted, unsupported mothers.

Chronic inflammation isn't always easy to diagnose, but can cause symptoms such as:

- constant fatigue and loss of energy, even after the simplest of activities
- brain fog
- bloating or changes in bowel habits
- joint pain and muscle stiffness
- headaches
- flare-ups of existing chronic conditions such as psoriasis, eczema, or dermatitis
- hair loss

Chronic inflammation can also increase your risk of developing autoimmune conditions, affect the thyroid, impact heart health, and lead to mental health problems.

Sleep disruption

Every woman's experience of pregnancy will differ. I often hear my patients complain of the insomnia of pregnancy or a new onset of heartburn, frequent urination, and anxiety, which all cause sleep disruptions. These, followed by the pressures and responsibilities of baby/toddler care, interfere with restful sleep leading to tiredness during the daytime. One study found that more than half of mothers worldwide reported poor sleep, so you're not alone.[2]

Why sleep matters

Many people think that you go to sleep and it's all part of one long stretch of sleep, when, in fact, sleep is a cycle made up of four different stages, all of equal importance:

- **Stage 1:** This is the drifting-off phase which lasts a few minutes. During this stage, the body relaxes and the heart rate and breathing slow down. This is when you can be easily woken up by light noises, like your baby crying.
- **Stage 2:** This is where you are drifting deeper. The body temperature drops and the brain, too, slows down. Most of our sleep state is in this phase, which helps to consolidate memory, and supports mental clarity and emotional regulation.
- **Stage 3:** This signals deep sleep, which really allows the body to get into a nice relaxing and restorative state. This is where we heal.
- **Stage 4:** This is rapid eye movement (REM) sleep. The brain becomes active and we start to dream when we enter the REM stage.

These different stages cycle between windows of 90 and 120 minutes and, together, influence how well the body repairs itself from the experiences it's had during the day, impacts our memory, and helps to regulate our emotional health.

When to seek help

Sleep deprivation is common in motherhood, especially in the early months and years, but it can have serious long-term effects.

Things to watch out for include:

Physical signs

- frequent headaches
- weakened immune system: catching everything that's going round
- increased clumsiness: dropping things, bumping into things
- extreme fatigue: falling asleep throughout the day, unable to complete tasks
- difficulty losing weight
- cardiovascular issues: including changes to your blood pressure and heart rate, and palpitations

Mental and emotional signs

- thoughts of self-harm or harming your baby
- disordered thinking or hallucinations
- complete inability to function or care for your baby
- brain fog and forgetfulness: losing track of time, misplacing items
- mood swings and irritability: snapping at your loved ones
- increased anxiety or feelings of being overwhelmed: persistent sadness, lack of motivation

Behavioural signs

- dozing off at the drop of a hat or when feeding your baby
- difficulty concentrating on simple tasks or struggling to follow conversations
- relying heavily on caffeine to function
- feeling emotionally detached from your baby or family

If you are experiencing any of these signs or symptoms, it's important to ask for help – whether that's time for a nap, extra support from family or your partner, or an appointment with your doctor. Sleep deprivation isn't just exhausting; it can take a serious toll on your mental and physical well-being too.

Vitamin deficiencies

There are a number of common vitamin deficiencies (which mothers are more prone to as they can neglect their own nutritional requirements) which can lead to maternal fatigue.

Firstly – and this is the one I see most in my mum patients – is **iron** deficiency anaemia. Symptoms of this include:

- overwhelming exhaustion
- shortness of breath
- light-headedness
- cold hands and feet
- palpitations
- weakness
- pale skin

While diet can help replenish this loss (leafy greens, lean meats, lentils, beans, and nuts are all good sources of iron), often iron supplements are required. Your doctor will run investigations including blood tests so they can treat the underlying cause.

Another common deficiency is **vitamin D** deficiency. Where you are in the world will affect how much vitamin D your body makes from sunlight (I live in Scotland, so getting sunshine is a rarity!). We need vitamin D for everything in our body – for brain function, cardiovascular health, immunity, bone health … you name it! Low vitamin D can cause fatigue or painful, achy bones, make you prone to infections, and can even affect your mood. Sunlight exposure is the answer, but, for most of us, and especially if you are darker skinned, cover your skin for cultural reasons, or are housebound, we need to take vitamin D all year round. You need it throughout your pregnancy and beyond, and your children also need it. It's the only vitamin I advise people to buy and take. (The need for other supplements will vary depending on clinical needs.) You can get some sources of vitamin D from the diet – for example, oily fish and fortified foods – but it's never enough, so take a supplement to avoid this deficiency.

You may have heard of people talking about **omega-3 fatty acids** which you can get from many foods like oily fish (salmon, mackerel, tuna, herring, sardines), nuts, and seeds (flaxseeds, chia seeds). Weaving these nutrients into the everyday as if they are essential non-negotiable supplements makes it easier. Omega-3 deficiency can cause you to feel drained and can also impact your mood, contributing to conditions like postpartum depression.

B12 and folate deficiency is common and can cause all sorts of symptoms like extreme fatigue, aching joints and weakness, pins and needles, poorer memory, and brain fog. We need these vital vitamins to help with our cellular health. They form part of the building blocks for our nervous system and red blood cell production.

The good news is that you can get these vitamins in a healthy balanced diet. Eggs are a great source of vitamin B12 and folate, as are leafy greens.

Last but not least, is good old **magnesium**. It's the least spoken about mineral and not many people understand or appreciate how important it is, especially for mums! Magnesium is a calming, gentle mineral which helps over 300 different enzyme reactions in the body. It affects our energy, mood, sleep, and stress levels, and a deficiency can cause insomnia, muscle cramps, and brain fog. For mums, especially in the postpartum or toddler phase, or entering the perimenopause era, magnesium often becomes depleted right when it's needed most.

Bananas are a good source of magnesium and are super easy to add into the daily snack regime, as are nuts, such as almonds and walnuts. Leafy greens, dark chocolate, wholemeal bread, and magnesium bath salts are also great ways to top up on magnesium, as are topical magnesium sprays and creams. From regulating the nervous system and supporting deep restorative sleep to helping ease muscle aches and pains and regulating hormones, magnesium can really help.

If needed and on the advice of a medical professional, use supplements if you are truly deficient in particular vitamins.

Easy ways to add more vitamins into your diet

- Always keep a bag of walnuts in your bag to snack on.
- Soak almonds in water overnight (which can improve their digestibility and increase nutrient absorption), peel off the skin and enjoy as a snack.
- Sprinkle seeds on porridge or add them to overnight oats.
- Add eggs into rice, noodles, or pasta, or simply have a boiled egg every day as part of your lunch.
- Blitz leafy greens into juices or smoothies, or add to sauces when cooking.
- Add bananas and berries to your porridge or yoghurt, have them as an easy midday snack or add them to a post-workout shake.

The mental load

I have spoken a lot about the physical causes of maternal exhaustion, but I must focus now on the lesser known or understood cause of maternal fatigue, and that is the mental and emotional load. I love the term 'invisible labour': the constant planning, organizing, micromanaging, decision-making, multitasking (even when resting!) … the list goes on. This is not about complaining, this is just stating pure fact. One study found that mothers overwhelmingly carry this mental load, while dads often take a back seat – with mums managing seven in ten household tasks.[3] This invisible labour causes emotional fatigue, sometimes compassion fatigue, and, in worse cases, maternal burnout.

While tiredness may be down to lifestyle factors, as we've seen, there can be underlying health conditions causing the fatigue. If rest does not alleviate your fatigue or it starts to affect your quality of life and everyday tasks, you must speak to your doctor. If you are experiencing anxiety, depression, or other mood disorders, this also needs to be reviewed by your doctor. (See Chapter 7 for more on these conditions.)

It is crucial that we understand the causes and manifestations of maternal fatigue, and, importantly, find solutions to support mothers because persistent exhaustion has implications, not only on maternal health, but on relationships, the development of children, and long-term outcomes at work. However, generation after generation, mothers are expected to carry the load quietly – exhausted, under-resourced, and ignored – while systems built around productivity, not people, continue to fail them. Globally, and here in the UK, maternal burnout is linked to poorer mental and physical health, increased pressure on healthcare systems, and long-term impacts on family well-being. We're tired of being tired. And it's time we demanded better.

Addressing maternal fatigue involves a combination of lifestyle adjustments and support systems. In the sections below, I've outlined some tips for the different stages of motherhood so you can alleviate fatigue and take back control.

'I'm Constantly Shattered': The Baby Years

During pregnancy and postpartum, women experience less REM sleep and so it's a no-brainer we feel so foggy and unable to function at 100 per cent. Instead of those lovely long, restorative sleep cycles we massively took for granted pre-kids, mums now get naps, squeezing in a wee sleep here or there. However, these bursts of sleep do not serve us in the long term and lead to us feeling emotionally 'all over the place' – a phrase I hear all the time in my clinic, and I immediately know the issue when women say it.

Newborn sleep cycles are unpredictable and this is exhausting, so it's important to recruit help if possible – at night or during the day – so you can get periods of REM sleep when you can. If your fatigue persists, speak to your health visitor or doctor for some advice and guidance.

But what if you are getting the sleep and still feel exhausted? Why does this happen?

Firstly, it may be due to natural instincts – as a new mum, you are instinctively on high alert. Your protective sense is more active than ever and, without realizing it, you are constantly in a state of 'fight or flight'. This can co-exist alongside the love, joy, and calm that is simultaneously being felt, but Mama Bear is always at the ready: *What was that noise the baby just made? What does it mean? Are they OK? Are they hungry? That poo didn't look right! Let me google this ... argh now I'm worried it's something serious!* This makes it harder to fully reach those deep, restorative sleep states we explored earlier. The overstimulation of the brain in this phase is a real phenomenon and, alongside the continuous interruptions, it means you only enter the lighter sleep cycles during the night. You're not imagining your tiredness.

Secondly, we focus so much on milestones and the baby's 'firsts', we forget that, when we enter motherhood, we, too, experience a lot of 'firsts'. We have all had the odd sleepless night, but the fragmented and bitty sleep on repeat is a first. The night feeds, the endless nappy changes, the strange noises newborns make that keep us on edge, teething, the irregular and evolving baby sleeping patterns – they're all firsts. It's A LOT to adapt and constantly adjust to.

And finally, pregnancy and breastfeeding can deplete the body's nutrient stores. If any of the symptoms on page 42 resonated with you, it's important to ensure you get this checked out and focus on replenishing any vitamins and minerals as necessary.

The role of hormones in new mum fatigue

During pregnancy and the postpartum seasons, women go through major hormonal shifts which influence our energy levels. There are various hormones at play here:

- **Progesterone:** This increases during pregnancy and contributes to excessive sleepiness and fatigue – in that first trimester especially when all you want to do is sleep for hours! After birth, it drops dramatically, which can lead to feelings of exhaustion and irritability.
- **Oestrogen:** This helps to increase energy levels and rises during pregnancy, but also has a drastic fall after the baby is born and we are left feeling knackered again, with mood swings and a sense of 'What just happened?'
- **Cortisol:** More commonly known as the stress hormone, this increases and fluctuates during pregnancy and beyond to help the body cope and adapt with all the physiological stress it is experiencing. Cortisol keeps you up, active, restless, angsty, prepared, and alert, and interferes significantly with the regulation of the sleep cycle.
- **Oxytocin:** Commonly referred to as the love hormone, this is a gorgeous hormone as it helps us bond with our babies. However, it, too, can interfere with the quality of our sleep as it can cause postpartum emotional sensitivity leading to feeling more emotionally vulnerable and fragile with more frequent night wakings.
- **Prolactin:** This is another hormone involved during this phase. Its job is to help with milk production, but it can cause fatigue in breastfeeding mums who may be at risk of nutritional deficiencies like iron deficiency anaemia (see page 43).

If you have a pre-existing condition like diabetes, thyroid disease, PCOS, postural orthostatic tachycardia syndrome (POTS), chronic fatigue syndrome or ME, or Lyme disease (to name a few), the subsequent postpartum fatigue may be more prominent and prolonged. Some women develop hormonal conditions during pregnancy and require more support. We need to raise awareness about this group of women because they really struggle to feel seen and heard – please speak to your doctor if you have any of these conditions and are experiencing extreme postpartum fatigue. There IS support out there for you.

What you can do

- **Prioritize rest – everything else can wait:** Rest will look different to every mum depending on their circumstances. It could look like sleeping or napping on the sofa. It could be having a bath or handing your baby over to someone so you have protected sleep time. However it looks, consistent downtime and sleeping improve long-term feelings of restfulness.

- **Seek support – it takes a village:** Remember, you are not alone so don't feel worried about asking for help, whether that's from your partner, family members, trusted friends, or babysitters/nannies. This was the best thing I ever did when I was initially struggling with it all. Everyone around you can help in some way; you just have to ask them. Asking for help does not make you a bad mum. On the contrary, it makes you a stronger mum, a mum who is investing in her future self by prioritizing her own healthcare needs. Lean on other people and ask them to deliver food/prep meals/do the housework. All these simple things really make a difference in these early days and leave you time to focus on your baby, establish a routine that works for you (tip: read your baby, not the manuals!), and, importantly, get some rest.

- **Practise relaxation techniques:** I prescribe you to take ten deep breaths three times a day – morning, afternoon, and night-time before closing your eyes to sleep. The breath is powerful; it's free and yours to use as you please. There are, of course, lots of accessible, free online videos, podcasts, yoga classes, and meditation lessons to help relax you … Whatever it is that works for you to help you unwind, slot it into your schedule as a non-negotiable and ensure everyone knows it's mandatory. You'll soon notice the difference. For me, I keep it simple. I do the breathing exercise I just shared with you, stand barefoot on the grass while I have my coffee in the morning, and go for a walk with my dog in silence after work every evening – it helps me to clear my mind.

- **Speak to your doctor:** Within the first few months post-baby, you should start to feel more yourself. However, if you continue to feel tired all the time with no energy, if your mood is low or you're anxious, if you are experiencing any new pains, especially around the back and pelvis, or you have any issues with libido, intercourse, or incontinence – anything that is unusual for you – do not ignore it and speak to your doctor (we'll deep dive into issues 'down below' in the next chapter).

'My Toddler Is Exhausting Me': The Toddler Years

We are often led to believe that it's the newborn phase that is the tricky one and things settle after this … well, it was only after becoming a mother myself that I learnt that this is not so true!

Toddlerhood is a rollercoaster ride. As our little ones start to unfold into their own personalities, it's a period of rapid growth and development. While this is beautiful and joyous to watch, it can also be a challenging time as they learn to become more independent and test boundaries. At this stage, therefore, maternal exhaustion takes another form – mums of toddlers often feel physically, mentally, and emotionally drained, especially if they are trying to juggle other kids and work and everything else life is throwing at them.

Toddlers require constant attention and vigilance because they are here, there, and everywhere. They are curious beings who are exploring the world with all their senses. They love to run, jump, climb, and touch everything, and are essentially a walking, kind-of-talking hazard! As mums, we are always on high alert, assessing for danger, and unable to relax as a result. It's exhausting.

Mood swings aren't just emotions that adults feel; no – toddlers feel big feelings too, but have no fear or awareness of when or where to express them as they are learning about their emotional well-being. You can call them tantrums, meltdowns, or expressions of emotions, but when they happen, it often falls on the mother to help calm and regulate them.

The juggle is real

You have the toddler, maybe other kids, maybe a pet, the house, the partner, and then work on top of all of that. You have to find ways to manage all of it, with the self-made pressure to achieve perfection – but then you end up frustrated, exhausted, and questioning what's wrong with you when you don't manage it. The reality is nobody can do it all. This era is hard work. It can be mentally, emotionally, and physically draining, and it's totally normal to feel this way.

One mum I saw in clinic recently burst into tears as she described her evenings. She had a toddler clinging to her legs while her eldest needed help with homework, and dinner was bubbling over on the hob. 'I'm always being pulled in every direction, and there's never a moment to breathe,' she told me. This is the kind of exhaustion that doesn't make headlines, but it's so relatable to most of us mums, and it builds slowly. It's not just tiredness. It's a constant state of overdrive.

I remember returning to work after my kids were at this stage and trying to balance the demands of my job, my colleagues, and the workload, plus the teething, potty training, and constant need for attention at home – it was exhausting. Even when you're not physically with your child, your brain is still working overtime: *Are they OK in childcare? Have they eaten? Am I a bad mum for leaving them?* It's a constant mental hum, a never-ending soundtrack of mum guilt. And let's be honest, for many women, going back to work isn't really a choice. The financial pressure is real, especially with the rising cost of living. Lots of mums return full-time, not because it feels right, but because they have to, and that adds another layer of emotional weight to an already exhausting season.

At the time of writing, I have just come out of the toddler phase with my little girl and, having done this twice, I have realized I have become one of the best negotiators around. From getting out of bed, brushing teeth, getting dressed, and eating breakfast to what songs are on the school run playlist, bath time, dinner, and bed time shenanigans, EVERYTHING is a discussion and grounds for negotiation. The mental load that comes with doing this day in and day out while adulting, parenting other kids, and working just adds to the exhaustion.

Toddlers are quite messy people and if you feel like you are just a glorified maid to them, it's because you are. With crumbs all over the place, toys scattered everywhere, not to mention the never-ending laundry piles, cooking, and so on, it's easy to see why mums feel the burn. Added to this is the pressure to 'bounce back' to how we were before having the baby!

Now, don't get me wrong, none of us would switch it, because we love and adore our kids, but I think it is very healthy to validate this facet of motherhood.

I'm afraid there is no on/off button and you are on-call 24/7, but there are things you can do to prevent burning out and, more importantly, preserve your energy and capacity. It's all about implementing small changes and putting in place some strategies to make this phase more manageable in the hope that it lightens the mother load somewhat.

Know that this is all totally normal and just try to go with the flow and not let perfectionist standards take control. Some tasks and chores can be left, a good cry is healthy, and taking time out for you is a positive move.

What you can do

- **Acknowledge and validate your feelings:** It feels challenging because it IS challenging, but remind yourself daily that you're doing a great job. Tell yourself what you would tell a fellow mum friend – give yourself the same kindness and compassion you give to others.
- **Routine is your best friend:** Plan the week – I always write it out – and stick to it. Humans thrive on routine; toddlers even more so. Explain to your child what's next or what the day will look like so everyone is on board. You are the leader, so try not to lose control. It's also important to remember, though, that it's OK if things don't turn out as planned.
- **Boundaries are key:** Know your limits and help your toddler to learn theirs. Saying 'no' doesn't make you a bad mum; it teaches your child safety, respect, and emotional regulation. Boundaries give children the structure they need to feel secure and the space you need to breathe. You don't have to say 'yes' to every demand or fix every feeling; you're allowed to prioritize your own well-being too.

'I Feel So Overwhelmed': The School/ Peri/Menopause Years

I think it's so important to acknowledge the fact that many women feel fatigue way beyond the postpartum phase – this is the bit no doctor so far has warned us about! I have lost count of the hours and energy spent managing the children's school admin, extracurricular activities, social calendars, meal plans, homework, conflicts ... This is on top of managing and juggling my own work schedules and home life, all while trying to practise what I preach as a doctor and eat well, exercise, get sleep, and manage my stress levels. Can you relate?

Children from the age of five onwards grow into more independent, social, emotional, and cognitively complex beings. There is no rule book or 'how-to' guide that comes with our kids either (now, wouldn't that be helpful!), so we have to figure them out one step at a time. Most mothers will agree that while this is a colourful and beautiful season of life, it is also the steepest learning curve. You are expected to know it all without having a clue about what's next. They ask you questions and you have very few answers; you are constantly on high alert, winging it and hoping that your actions will somehow result in raising the children you dreamt you'd raise. Oh, the pressure is real, isn't it?

I know I am not alone in this. The scenario I share is a collective daily effort most mothers experience; some more than others. If you are a single parent with limited childcare support, it's even more challenging. This is not a complaint or a moan – it's just the reality of maternal lifestyles today. We have to recognize and validate it.

Mothers are often the child's primary comfort blankets. We want to ensure our kids feel seen and heard and, over time, this can lead to compassion fatigue, especially if you are caring for others too – whether that's other children, children with additional needs, or relatives. Nobody warns you about the constant decision-making that comes with these years, which can also contribute to the overwhelm. This is rarely acknowledged and there is little awareness about the phenomenon known as 'decision fatigue', coined by Roy Baumeister, which takes its toll if left unmanaged and unsupported over a period of time.[4] From big decisions to tiny ones – and not to mention the endless to-do lists – many mothers find switching off difficult, which impacts the quality and quantity of sleep they get and triggers anxiety and stress.

For many women, the reality is that not only are you managing the transitions your children are going through, you may also be going through changes yourself … If you are a mother in your late 30s or 40s and you feel like you're losing your mind, you're absolutely not. You're not making it up. You're not 'going crazy'. It might be that you're perimenopausal. While menopause is defined as the point 12 months after your last period, the years leading up to that – known as perimenopause – can cause a shift in how many women think and feel. It can impact physical, mental, and emotional well-being due to the fluctuating levels of key hormones like oestrogen and progesterone.

Much to the surprise of many women, perimenopause often begins in the late 30s to early 40s. In the UK, about 50 per cent of women begin to notice perimenopausal symptoms (such as mood swings, sleep issues, and irregular cycles) by the age of 44 or 45, and 85 per cent experience physical or psychological symptoms at this time.[5] This phase can last for up to 10 years and can take many women on a hormonal rollercoaster, which impacts all aspects of a women's body – her mood, energy, skin, digestion … everything! And, if you are a new mum during this time, it can significantly add to maternal exhaustion.

One of the most common things women going through the perimenopause tell me is how unpredictable the symptoms can be. No two women will experience the same symptoms and so it can be challenging to manage. In tandem with the unpredictable fatigue, this can make for quite a difficult time if issues are not identified and treated adequately.

When you are already feeling tired and not getting enough restful and uninterrupted sleep, the nuisance of peri/menopausal hot flushes keeping you up can really tip you and your sanity over the edge. Alongside this, hormonal fluctuations can impact your energy levels and sleep patterns, and trigger feelings of unexplained anxiety, mood swings, irritability, and a loss in sense of 'self'. If you are already experiencing this as a mother to young kids, peri/ menopause can really heighten those feelings.

Another common symptom of perimenopause is brain fog, which can be distressing as often patients express anxiety or fear about whether they have dementia. If you've ever experienced brain fog, you will know that it is quite frightening. However, if you are already a mother carrying most of the visible and invisible load of the household, it's hard to differentiate what's causing what. The brain is a finite resource and there's only so much you can expect of it before it starts to show signs that it's overwhelmed. There is more on the reality of brain fog in Chapter 6.

Sadly, due to the historic lack of education and awareness, many mothers don't even know they are going through perimenopause. They can be gas-lit by family members, colleagues, and even medical experts that it's 'all in their head' or just part of motherhood when, in fact, there are significant physiological shifts happening within their body, causing discomfort in their own skin and making them question their sense of identity. The most important thing anyone can do is believe a woman when she says 'something is not right'. Never let anyone minimize or disregard your feelings.

While it might feel like you need to do more and more as the needs of your children grow, I believe the secret is actually in simplifying it right down. Instagram mums will show you curated highlight reels on how to be the 'perfect' parent in today's world. There are always a million hacks, tips, and tricks you could try, but, even with those, all this extra consumption of content can feel a lot. It can also put you in the comparison trap. Instead, think of what mums in the olden days would've done. I find this usually helps me. Modern-day parenting has become too much of a 'task' when, actually, we need to reconnect with our unique and natural flows. You don't need to go everywhere and ensure your children are attending every event/party/activity/trip. Be selective and know that it's OK to say no. Kids get overwhelmed too and families need 'downtime' together in today's fast-paced life. In fact, research has shown that it is in the quiet, pondering, 'boring' moments that our brains become alive and start to imagine, wonder, dream, and create.[6] There's a magic and power in stillness for us all.

I know these years can feel challenging, but remind yourself that you are absolutely doing an incredible job and there are things you can do to lighten the load.

What you can do

- **Take a moment:** It seems simple, but among the chaos, we often forget the impact that taking just 5 minutes (in whatever way we can) to gather our thoughts can have to help recalibrate, clear the mind, and boost energy. That might be stepping outside, looking up at the sky, and taking some deep breaths (moments of mindfulness like this are really calming for the nervous system), or making a cup of tea and sitting down – whatever works for you.
- **Speak to your family, friends, and colleagues about how you are feeling:** Don't bottle it up. Trust me, you are not alone, and by opening up you will find support and help so you can feel better.
- **Prioritize sleep:** This is paramount when it comes to peri/menopause. Setting a consistent bedtime and screen-free evening routine will help, as will the addition of things like magnesium supplements/bath soak (magnesium supports the nervous system, helps regulate the sleep hormone melatonin, and promotes muscle relaxation, all of which can make it easier to fall into a deeper, more restorative sleep – see page 44).

Punam's Prescription

Do a self-audit

Get yourself a notebook or use your phone Notes app and, for a minimum of two weeks, ask yourself these two questions first thing every morning:

1. Do I feel tired this morning? Yes / No
2. How are my energy levels this morning? 30 per cent / 60 per cent / 90 per cent

I've simplified it right down because I know you don't have time for anything more complicated, so there's no need to write essays if that's not your thing, but this simple audit is a fantastic way to get a snapshot of how tired you really feel and stay ahead of sleep deprivation. It is also handy to talk to your doctor if you're at a stage where you need to take action to reclaim your sleep cycle.

Take 10

I prescribe you 10 minutes in the morning, afternoon, and evening to lighten the exhaustion and reset:

- Take 10 minutes in the morning for journaling to create capacity in your mind (I call this 'the Mum Dump'). You can use your Notes app on your phone or a notebook. See it like a loo break and get it all out. Nobody else needs to see or read it, but you will find that, suddenly, you will have a bit more headspace and capacity to think.
- Take 10 minutes in the afternoon to do some movement, such as stretching – there are lots of apps out there to help with this.

- Take 10 minutes in the evening for something that sparks joy to recalibrate. This could be reading, having a quiet cuppa, grounding, dancing ... whatever works for you.

Maintain a balanced diet

Mums can often fall victim to cutting corners when it comes to eating. Maybe you're exhausted and don't have the energy to cook for yourself so will eat the scraps off your child's plate and be done. It's time to change that. Food *is* energy and, if you want to feel energized, you need to fuel yourself with a healthy, balanced diet. What you make so lovingly for your child, give yourself that same love. Don't wait until after your child has gone to bed to sit down and eat – it will likely be later than is healthy anyway. Eat those veggies, and the broccoli trees! And while I have you – take the vitamins too. Mothers often forget to mother themselves.

From weaning to beyond, get into the habit of cooking and eating together as a family – it has so many benefits (for both adults and children), including feeling happier and having a chance to connect and unwind with loved ones.[7] There is even evidence to suggest that social connection supports gut health.[8] And let's not forget that it also teaches children valuable life skills, such as table manners and healthy eating habits. In contrast, eating late, knackered, while doing chores or watching the telly isn't restorative in quite the same way (but OK on occasion!).

In addition, as kids get older, getting them involved in the kitchen and clean up can ease your load and help their learning.

Move that body – every movement counts!

Start simple and build the habit to move for yourself every single day – nothing complex or fancy required. We mums don't have much time, but even a simple stretch helps to induce those feelings of calm. Move the neck and shoulders, which is where we hold all that tension, bend and feel the stretch along your back, reach for your toes and the ceiling, and take some nice deep breaths. Stretch to your own ability and seek specific guidance from a physiotherapist or personal trainer.

Even on the days when you're so unbearably tired, get some steps in, do some squats, or climb some stairs, and try do it with the kids if you can. I walk to get my patients from the waiting room and race my kids from the car to the school gates – it all adds up. You don't need energy to start – movement helps create it. Trust me, it'll make you sleep better!

Final Thoughts

If you are experiencing any of the signs and symptoms of maternal fatigue we've covered in this chapter, it's time to get help to sort this out. You do not have to live like this forever. As women, the odds are already often stacked against us, but there is help and support to manage this and get you feeling more energized and like yourself again.

In case you're wondering, I too have been there and often feel exhausted. Have I got it all figured out? No. Am I also a work in progress? Yes. I practise all the things I advise in this chapter and, some days, I am fully recharged with energy and super-efficient at using it, but, other days, I'm just managing at 50 per cent. What's different now to when I burnt out a few years ago is that I can recognize the signs when I'm flagging and operating suboptimally and know what steps I can take to prevent that maternal burnout before it happens (more on that in Chapter 8).

CHAPTER 3

'Nothing Looks or Feels Normal Down There'

MANAGING TEARS, PROLAPSE, INCONTINENCE, AND EVERYTHING IN BETWEEN

As a medical student and later a junior doctor, I attended and assisted in many births. I got to be there for all the stages of labour – the messy and the beautiful bits – but then I never saw the woman or her family again. I dealt with the immediate complications, but always wondered how they impacted the patient in the long term. It's one of the reasons I decided to become a GP because while working in a hospital is exciting – and I enjoyed the adrenaline rush that came from problem-solving in emergency situations – I love people and their journeys more. I like to get to know my patients and review and manage their long-term outcomes.

As a younger GP, I also never got to fully appreciate how women were healing after childbirth because very few would come forward to share their birth stories. Sadly, women often experience complications 'down below' after birth, but these are not openly discussed because they are considered 'taboo'. Birth experiences remain hidden beneath the surface due to fear of how they might be received, feelings of shame, or for cultural reasons. The Royal College of Obstetricians & Gynaecologists

(RCOG), for example, found that 69 per cent of women had not spoken to anyone in the NHS about their pelvic floor health – we need to change this.[1]

Of course, it also doesn't help that there is no global, universally mandated system for postnatal care – and so postnatal assessments and who provides them varies from country to country. In the UK, for example, aside from the usual basic postnatal screening questions at the six-week check which go along the lines of, 'How are you?', 'All healing well?', and 'Have you thought about contraception?', no specifics about 'issues down below' are discussed (unless there's a serious problem). Until I had my first baby and subsequent complications, I hadn't appreciated just how much of a failed system we have.

Looking around the world, it really is fascinating how dramatically the quality of postnatal care varies. The World Health Organization (WHO) recommends a minimum of four postnatal check-ins in the first six weeks after birth, covering both physical and emotional recovery, breastfeeding support, and reviews of complications. The reality, however, is that millions of women worldwide are discharged from the labour ward and then largely left to cope alone.

In the US, most new mums receive just one routine visit at six weeks. In Australia, care is also patchy and often depends on a postcode lottery or private access. In contrast, I look to countries like Sweden and Norway, and they take a much more holistic approach, offering regular home visits by midwives or health visitors, and generous parental leave that supports both mother and father bonding and healing. If I look across to south Asia and India, postnatal care varies hugely. Urban areas offer better access, but many women in rural areas receive little to no follow-up. Even in high-income nations, few meet the WHO gold standard, and that gap between what mums should get and what they actually get is too big to ignore.

Added to this, women's experiences are often not medically validated, which means that they suffer silently, believing their incisional or pelvic pains, sexual discomfort, urinary or bowel incontinence, or fear and avoidance of further essential gynaecological procedures are all normal when they're not.

The physical changes we experience after birth is one of those areas that can really hold us back from feeling like our best boss selves – whatever stage of life we're at. But you deserve answers, support, and to feel confident in your body – always. It's time to have the conversation most of us never had: the one about what really happens down there – and what can actually help – because it can feel really isolating, especially when no one talks about these complications post-birth.

In this chapter, we'll look at everything from birth recovery through to perimenopause, and every leaky, sore, and slightly embarrassing stage in between, because the truth is that motherhood does change everything and that's OK. We just need to be informed about it. We'll talk about the spectrum of physical scars that birth can cause, stress and urge incontinence, the different types of prolapse, and whether the discharge you're having is normal or not. We'll also look at how some of these issues can linger in later life and how you can still heal even years down the line. Even though they are not directly linked to issues 'down below', I'm also going to touch on breast changes here because it's another physical change that so many women are worried about and I want to ensure you are as informed as possible when it comes to your body.

Before we dive in, I think it's important that you first understand that giving birth – however that has been – is a major event, so it's normal to come away from it with a changed pelvic area. Complications 'down below' are part and parcel of having a baby, but they can get better and should not persist throughout your lifetime.

What's Normal After Birth?

Looseness or laxity is extremely common after vaginal birth. This is because the vaginal walls, pelvic floor muscles, and connective tissues can stretch significantly over several months. It is therefore normal for it to take several months for things to settle or, as some would say, 'bounce back'. You might feel more 'open', less supported, or that there is less resistance when inserting a tampon or even during intercourse. These sensations are totally normal in the early postpartum days and, for many, they gradually improve over time and with pelvic floor exercises (see page 90 for guidance on this).

Other common sensations include:

- a heaviness or dragging from the vagina, especially towards the end of the day (though this can be a sign of prolapse – we'll talk more about this later in the chapter)
- passing wind from the vagina (vaginal flatulence) due to changes in pelvic floor tone
- mild incontinence – especially when laughing, sneezing, or coughing

If you've had a C-section, it's completely normal to feel sore and tender around the wound for several days to weeks. Most women require regular pain relief for at least the first few weeks. It can take anything from eight to twelve weeks to six to twelve months for your body to heal properly.

'Lochia' – the term we give to immediate discharge post-birth which is a mix of blood, mucus, and even some tissue from the womb – is also typical for women after both a vaginal delivery and a C-section.

Most of these symptoms are temporary. However, there are some symptoms that warrant further investigation, which I've listed in the box that follows.

When to seek help

If you experience any of the following symptoms, seek medical help as soon as possible:

- pain during or bleeding after sex
- a sudden change in vaginal discharge
- any bulging from the vagina
- burning, dryness, or pain in the vagina
- persistent incontinence
- numbness or pressure that persists
- any pain or foul smell from the vaginal/vulval area

'Is My Wound/Scar Meant to Look Like This?'

How you choose to deliver your baby is your choice and there is no right or wrong way to birth (though I appreciate we don't always have a choice if something doesn't go to plan). There are, however, births that increase our risk of having complications, which include episiotomies, instrumental deliveries, and C-sections. Where interventions have taken place, you have a higher risk of infections, bleeding, or complications with subsequent healing and scarring, so it's important that you know what to watch out for.

Vaginal births

According to the RCOG, up to nine in every ten first-time mothers who have a vaginal birth experience some form of perineal trauma which can range from small cuts to significant tears.[2] However, many of these women are sent home simply with mild pain relief, a leaflet, and a belief that this is 'normal'. It's not.

It can feel scary if nobody explains what happened or what it all means, so let's break it down.

Perineal tears
There are four types of perineal tears:

1. **First-degree tear:** This involves just the skin around the vaginal opening. It's usually small and does not need any stitches.It heals on its own and quickly, usually within a couple of weeks. It feels like a sting or graze, especially when you pee, but, in general, it causes no long-term complications.
2. **Second-degree tear:** This involves the skin and the muscle of the perineum. It always requires stitches, which are dissolvable, and healing takes around two to four weeks. It's sore – and can be when sitting or during sex for a while, but most women recover well and fully.
3. **Third-degree tear:** This is more serious as it can extend from the perineal muscles into the muscle around the anus. Third-degree tears are further classified as 3A, 3B, or 3C depending on how much of the sphincter muscle has torn. Third-degree tears require surgical intervention and healing takes longer, usually six weeks or more. It is essential that women with third-degree tears have input from a specialist physiotherapist as this type of tear can lead to bowel urgency or incontinence if not managed well.
4. **Fourth-degree tear:** This is the most severe and, thankfully, rare. It goes through the anal sphincter, which is what controls the opening and closing of the anus when we poo, and requires surgical repair and takes longer to heal. There is an increased risk of long-term bowel control issues with this type of tear and so early intervention and combined care from different health professionals is essential.

Tearing during birth is very common, especially for first-time vaginal births. If you've had an assisted delivery, such as forceps or ventouse, there's a higher risk of third- or fourth-degree tears.

How perineal tears affect women

- pain when sitting or walking
- pain when opening bowels
- leaking wind or stool
- fear of exercise
- avoidance of sex
- heavy, dragging pelvic sensations
- embarrassment and distress

Women often suffer silently, but there is help and support available, so please see your family doctor if you are affected by any of these issues.

Tearing isn't your fault and you are not alone if you feel scared, sore, or just unsure of what the long-term risks could be. However, knowing that you have the right to request intervention and good-quality care is empowering.

Episiotomies

During vaginal birth, surgical cuts may be made in the perineum (the area between the vagina and anus) – known as episiotomies. These are common and are a decision made by your labour team if they feel there will be any difficulty getting your baby out and so the vaginal opening is enlarged by making an incision. Episiotomies are also carried out if there is a concern that there could be a greater, less controlled natural tear which could cause severe bleeding. If you have had an episiotomy, it is horrible, and I'm sorry you had to go through it.

There are several things you can do to help heal your episiotomy or tear:

- **Keep it clean:** Rinse the area gently with warm water after using the toilet to help prevent infection. Pat dry with a soft towel or let it air dry. Avoid using soaps, bubble baths, or wipes, as these can irritate healing skin.
- **Don't overdo things:** Be careful not to push yourself too hard – rest is essential after birth.
- **Stay well-hydrated and add extra fibre to your diet:** Soft stools are key. If needed, your doctor may recommend laxatives.
- **Soothe the area:** A sitz bath (a warm shallow bath) or cool packs work well to reduce the swelling and inflammation, and relieve any discomfort.
- **Talk about it:** Too often, women are told to just 'get on with it' after birth, but it's OK and normal to feel sore, vulnerable, or even emotionally shaken. Don't suffer in silence – speak to your midwife, doctor, or health visitor if you're in pain, worried about healing, or if sex feels uncomfortable. These wounds are physical and emotional, and being heard can be an important part of healing.

When to seek help

There are some things to look out for if you've had an episiotomy or natural tear:

- **Increasing pain:** Soreness is expected, but it should feel manageable with pain relief. If the pain is worsening instead of improving, it may be a sign of infection or poor healing.
- **Other signs of infection:** These include redness, swelling, feeling hot around the wound, pus or yellow/green discharge, foul-smelling discharge, fevers, and chills.
- **Wound opening (known as wound dehiscence):** If stitches

are coming apart or it looks like there is a gap, get
it looked at sooner rather than later.
- **Pain when peeing or opening your bowels.**
- **Painful intercourse.**
- **Hard lumps around the tear.**

If you are experiencing any of these, please see your doctor
and get checked out.

Caesarean sections

When you have a C-section, an incision is made across the lower
abdomen just above the pubic area. While your wound will be
visible externally, many layers of tissue, muscle, and fat had to be
cut through and stitched back up during the surgery – and this
usually takes about three months to heal. It's also important to
remember that while a C-section can be life-saving, it can still be
traumatic. If a woman felt forced into it or it was poorly explained,
it can lead to psychological distress.

It's often not appreciated that a C-section is major abdominal
surgery – mums are sent home, with minimal aftercare,
with a newborn, and every circumstance imaginable that
will hinder their healing process: they will have little sleep,
questionable nutritional replenishment, may be breastfeeding,
and will need to contort themselves into all sorts of positions
to cater for their baby's comforts, all at the expense of their
own recovery.

Healing from a C-section is not just about resting, it's about
doing everything you can to aid the recovery process:

- **Keep the area clean and dry:** You don't need fancy
  products; simple cooled boiled water will do the job, but
  no scrubbing or picking.

- **Avoid straining:** Try to not lift anything heavier than your baby for at least six weeks.
- **Consider additional support:** Wearing a supportive postpartum band or high-waisted underwear will help to gently hold in the area.
- **Reduce pressure on the wound:** When coughing, laughing, or sneezing, try holding a pillow or cushion over your belly to help ease the pressure.
- **Stay hydrated:** This will help support tissue repair and avoid constipation, which can add pressure to the wound when straining.
- **Ensure you are eating a healthy diet:** Try adding in turmeric to help with the healing as it has powerful anti-inflammatory properties.
- **Try scar massage:** This can help after six weeks.

When to seek help

While most C-section wounds heal well, there are some important things to look out for:

- **Signs of infection:** These include redness that's spreading around the incision site, swelling or warmth around the wound, pus or foul-smelling discharge, fever or chills, or pain that is increasing rather than steadily improving.
- **Opening of the wound (dehiscence):** Stitches may come apart or there may be a visible gap and/or fluid leaking from the wound.
- **Persistent pain that doesn't ease or becomes worse.**
- **Lumps:** These may feel bumpy or have fluid or blood in them.
- **Unusual bleeding from the wound.**
- **Hernia:** This is where an organ may pop through tissue, causing a bulge.

- **Numbness or tingling around the belly area:** Due to the nature of the surgery, sometimes nerves can be damaged during the procedure, which can cause numbness or tingling – this is not a nice feeling! Sometimes the numbness can be temporary, but it can be permanent.

If you experience any of these symptoms, do not ignore them and speak to your family doctor right away.

The long-term impact of birth

We often think of wounds healing as the end of the story, but, for some women, it's just the beginning of ongoing symptoms that aren't talked about enough. As your body heals from birth, whether from a tear, an episiotomy, or a C-section, it's normal for scar tissue to form. But, sometimes, this tissue develops into adhesions: internal bands that stick organs or tissues together. These can cause persistent pain in the pelvis or lower abdomen, painful periods, discomfort during sex, changes to bowel habits, and even reduced mobility in some cases. Once formed, adhesions don't tend to go away on their own and, in severe cases, may require surgical treatment.

Another condition that can arise after pregnancy or uterine procedures is adenomyosis, where the lining of the womb starts to grow into the muscle wall of the uterus. It can cause heavy, painful periods, deep pelvic pain, fatigue, and pain during sex. Many women go undiagnosed for years, assuming their symptoms are just part of 'normal' womanhood. Similarly, endometriosis – where womb-like tissue grows outside the uterus – can cause a wide range of symptoms, such as intense period pain, bloating, fatigue, bowel issues, and fertility struggles. Both conditions are often misunderstood, misdiagnosed, or dismissed altogether.

In perimenopause and menopause, falling oestrogen levels reduce the elasticity and strength of tissues throughout the body, and the pelvic floor is no exception. Muscles, ligaments, and connective tissues that may have held up well for years after childbirth can suddenly become weaker or less supportive. This means that injuries from pregnancy or birth, even those from decades earlier, can start to reappear or worsen. For some women, this is the first time they start to experience symptoms like vaginal heaviness, bladder leakage, painful sex, or pelvic pain, and it's often the first time they open up about a difficult or traumatic birth experience they've kept quiet about for years. The body is finally saying what words never could.

This is something I see regularly in clinic: women in their 40s or 50s suddenly coming forward with symptoms that trace back to tears that didn't heal properly, forceps deliveries, long labours, or C-section scars that never quite felt right. Until now, they've just got on with it, but the hormonal shift of perimenopause strips away the scaffolding their body has relied on. What's left is the unspoken legacy of birth that was never addressed at the time.

If you're experiencing pain that's affecting your quality of life, it matters. You matter. If something doesn't feel right, keep pushing for answers. Track your symptoms and take them to your family doctor. And if you're not being heard, ask again. You're not being difficult, you're being thorough, and that's exactly what your body deserves.

What you can do

- **Don't suffer in silence:** Motherhood conditions us to ignore ourselves – we are always at the bottom of the to-do list. But don't be shy of asking a doctor, nurse, or health visitor to have a look at your tear or C-section wound if you're worried – don't put it off. It's OK to ask, 'Can you check my stitches?', for example, for that peace of mind. If things haven't got better in six months, make an appointment with your family doctor rather than worrying about it. And, whatever you do, don't rely on Dr Google!

- **Trust your instincts:** You know your body best – if something doesn't feel right, even if it's 'just a niggle', get it checked.

- **See a pelvic health physiotherapist:** If you're dealing with pain, heaviness, leakage, or anything that just doesn't feel quite right 'down below' after birth, a pelvic health physio is the person to see. These are specialist physiotherapists trained in assessing and treating issues with the pelvic floor, abdominal wall, and surrounding muscles. They can support your recovery after birth trauma, help retrain weak or overactive pelvic muscles, and offer expert advice on movement, breathing, and exercises tailored to your body. If you are in the UK, speak to your GP to request an NHS referral – or if you're seeing someone privately, make sure they're registered with the Chartered Society of Physiotherapy (CSP) or Pelvic, Obstetric and Gynaecological Physiotherapy (POGP). If you don't have access to a physio or time is tight, you're not alone – but you still deserve support. Many maternity units now offer online workshops or leaflets with safe postnatal recovery advice – ask your health visitor or doctor about what's available in your area.

'I Only Sneezed – Why Am I Leaking?'

During the birth of my first child, a series of mistakes and problems along the way during a long labour resulted in an emergency forceps delivery causing a 3B tear (see page 66). This is when 50 per cent of the anal sphincter (the muscles that control pooing and farting – there's no nicer way to explain it!) tears. We get told that your dignity goes out the door when giving birth, but this took things to a whole other level for me. Everything else was an openly talked about complication of birth – we bleed, we still look pregnant and huge after birth, we have leaky boobs – but we don't poo ourselves ... or do we?

Childbirth – especially via instrumental deliveries or if you have a prolonged labour or a large baby – can cause weakening of the pelvic floor. After birth, women often experience:

- urgency
- leaking when coughing or sneezing
- incomplete emptying of the bladder or bowels
- urinary retention

By three months post-birth, one in three women report urinary incontinence and one in six have anal incontinence, but instead of being routinely offered support and recovery, many women are left to manage their symptoms in silence.[3] These are not minor issues – they are serious public health failures in my opinion, but they remain under-treated because women have historically been taught to laugh it off, 'just do their Kegels', and get on with it.

Here's the kicker: if men leaked urine every time they laughed, sneezed, or jumped, or if their underwear was streaked with faeces or they couldn't get to the toilet in time, there would be rows and rows of shelves stacked with products dedicated to solving it. We would be bombarded with advertisements raising awareness, but when it comes to us women? 'It's just part of having kids,' we're told. But I'm here to change that.

In order to understand why some women leak after birth, let's get back to basics and look at what the pelvic floor actually is. This is the term we use to describe the group of muscles that sit like a hammock at the base of your pelvis. Their job is to help support your bladder, your bowel, and your womb. They're key for controlling your pee, wind, and poo, but what very few people realize is that they're also super important for posture, core strength, and even sex. So, when they are not working well, you feel it in more ways than one. Pregnancy, vaginal birth, hormonal loss during the peri/menopause, chronic constipation, chronic coughing, and even heavy lifting can cause these muscles to over-stretch, weaken, or even tear, and that's when you can develop:

- **Stress incontinence:** This causes leaking of urine when you cause any strain like coughing, jumping, running, or sneezing. Just over 20 per cent of women experience this after childbirth.[4]
- **Urge incontinence:** This is when you get a sudden and intense need to pee, and sometimes it may even be followed by a leak. This often starts in our 30s or 40s when hormonal shifts start and contribute to the weakening of our pelvic floor muscles. Common triggers include running water, cold weather, exercise, or even unlocking the front door.
- **Bowel incontinence:** Also known as faecal incontinence, this is when you have difficulty controlling your bowel movements, leading to the involuntary leakage of stool (solid or liquid) or, in some cases, gas. It ranges from occasional small leaks when passing wind, to more noticeable loss of stool that can interfere with daily life. Bowel incontinence happens because the muscles and nerves that control the anus and pelvic floor can be weakened or injured during pregnancy and birth, especially if there was significant tearing, prolonged labour, instrumental delivery (forceps/vacuum), or sphincter injury. These symptoms can be distressing and affect quality of life, but they are treatable, especially when addressed early with pelvic health support.

You can have one or all of these types of incontinence, and it can be deeply frustrating, embarrassing, worrying, and debilitating, stopping you from planning trips and activities.

I often see mums (I might be guilty of this myself) doing the 'just in case pee' before every school run, work meeting, or travel. We start doing things like not drinking water in case we can't find a toilet or map out a day where toilet stops are part of the itinerary. Sound familiar? And it's not just the bladder. For some women, bowel control becomes a hidden stress. I've spoken to mums who avoid coffee or certain foods before leaving the house, or who always carry spare underwear or pads just in case. These are practical adaptations, but they also speak to the quiet, often unspoken impact childbirth can have on our pelvic health.

While I totally get it, I have to tell you that this is the worst thing we can do to ourselves because, in doing all of the above, we are actually handing all power to our bladders and bowels. If left unmanaged from the get-go, the problems only worsen, especially when the hormonal changes that come with perimenopause kick in (see below for more on this).

I promise you, I know how it can feel because I've lived with it too. My son is 11 at the time of writing and I still work on my pelvic floor. It's not a quick fix – recovery takes time, but healing is absolutely possible. The earlier we start our pelvic floor rehab, the better because it gives us the best chance to heal, to feel in control again, and to get back to life before things get more complicated or start affecting our everyday confidence.

When incontinence lingers

I have heard many clinicians over my 20 years as a doctor say that perimenopause is 'just an age thing'. I would argue instead that it's childbirth catching up on us. Nobody warns you it's coming and, suddenly, hormones start fluctuating, which impacts every part of us, and we're launched into a whole new transitional phase – boom, we're in perimenopause. So many women in their 40s and 50s message me saying, 'I've started leaking; is that normal?' And while it's not normal, it's sadly very common. One patient I saw recently told me she'd been 'managing' a bit of bladder leakage ever since her second baby by doing pelvic floor squeezes now and then, avoiding certain workouts, and always knowing where the nearest loo was. She never made a fuss. But now in her mid-40s, she's started leaking during everyday things like walking the dog, laughing too hard, or getting up from a chair. 'It's like everything I've been brushing off for years has suddenly caught up with me,' she said. She thought she was doing something wrong. In reality, her hormones were shifting and the oestrogen that once gave her pelvic tissues elasticity and support was starting to fall. This wasn't her failing, it was the result of years of quiet compromises, made after birth, now colliding with the physiological changes of perimenopause.

What the science says

As levels of the hormone oestrogen start to drop during the perimenopause, it leads to GSM, causing tissue thinning in the pelvic area (see page 29). These changes mean you've got even less support down there and therefore more chances of leaking. Sometimes, this weakening can also lead to prolapse, which we'll discuss in just a bit. If that wasn't enough, to make things trickier, the bladder itself becomes more sensitive with hormonal changes too, so you might feel sudden urges to pee, you might be peeing more often, or you might start waking up in the night to pass urine, and it's not all just about the muscles. During peri/menopause, your whole system can change – your hormones fluctuate, your weight changes, and your sleep and energy levels fall – and this puts extra pressure on the pelvic floor too. So, you might find that you're leaking when you laugh, sneeze, or exercise, or that you're rushing to the loo and not quite making it on time.

I'm here to tell you that it's never too late to start taking care of your pelvic floor, so even if it's been years since you had your baby, please don't just pad it or ignore it. You should feel confident to talk about it – and get the help you deserve.

If you leak when you cough, move, or laugh, your body is asking for help. Don't ignore it! The key here is knowing that you have got options, you've got support, and you don't have to just live with it. If something feels off, please speak up, because this is treatable and you can feel confident in your body again.

What you can do

- **Do your pelvic floor exercises (also known as Kegels):** Pelvic floor weakness is a common cause of incontinence, so these are a must. However, it's important that you learn how to do them correctly – studies show that 50 per cent of women perform Kegels incorrectly.[5] See my Prescription on page 90 for more guidance on this.

- **Speak to your doctor:** Pelvic floor rehabilitation is one of the first steps, but there are lots of reasons women leak: hormonal changes (pregnancy/perimenopause/menopause), birth trauma, prolapse, nerve damage, chronic constipation, or chronic coughing, to name but a few. That's why support and assessment are so important. Try to get to the root cause of the problem. Bladder medications can help calm that overactive urge and, if a prolapse is involved, then pessaries can offer support and relief too. You might also want to consider hormone replacement therapy (HRT) if you are eligible. Vaginal oestrogen can help restore tissue strength and support, and it's a game changer for many women going through peri/menopause. In some cases, for some women, surgery might be an option, but it's usually considered alongside other treatments, not instead of them.

- **Retrain your bladder:** This really works, but patience and consistency are key! Start by delaying urination in small increments – for example, if you go every 30 minutes, try holding off for 35 minutes and then 40 and so on. You can also try some exercises to suppress the urge like sitting still and breathing slowly while contracting your pelvic floor (three to five squeezes). This relaxes the nervous system and allows the bladder to calm down. If things don't improve, there are medications that are effective and work well, such as antimuscarinics (for example, Solifenacin) which relaxes the oversensitive and hyperactive bladder, as well as beta-3 agonists (for example, Mirabegron) which lets the bladder hold more urine. These medications are safe and effective but are also under-prescribed.
- **Tweak your lifestyle:** Try cutting down on caffeine, especially after 2pm as it is a diuretic and can make symptoms worse. If you struggle with constipation, review your diet and/ or get medical help as this can put additional pressure on the bladder and bowel. Losing weight can also reduce pressure on the pelvic floor and make a big difference.

'It Feels Like Something Is Falling Out Down Below'

Remember, your pelvic floor is like a hammock which supports your bladder, your womb, and your bowel. When it is strong, it holds everything up. However, when it is damaged (for example, during childbirth), it starts to sag and so everything that is resting on it starts to sag down too.

A pelvic organ prolapse (known as POP) happens when the muscles and connective tissues of the pelvic floor become stretched or weakened, meaning that the organs within the pelvis can shift from their usual position to other areas, sometimes even outside of the vagina.

There are different types of prolapses. The common ones include:

- **Bladder prolapse (cystocele):** This is where the bladder bulges into the front wall of the vagina.
- **Bowel prolapse (rectocele):** This is where the rectum presses down into the back vaginal wall.
- **Womb (uterine) prolapse:** This is where the uterus comes down into or out of the vaginal canal.

A prolapse can cause leaking or a pressure sensation. Women often describe it as 'heaviness' or a feeling that they are dragging something in their pelvis. A bulge may be seen or felt during an examination. Women may find inserting tampons difficult or find it hard to fully empty their bowel or bladder. It can feel like something is falling out, sex may be painful, and, in worst cases, lower back pain may develop and become a chronic problem.

Prolapse can affect everything from sex, exercise, and continence to mental well-being, body image, and confidence. Despite the unnecessary shame and stigma that is often linked to prolapse, it is extremely common. Studies indicate that up to 50 per cent of women will develop some kind of POP over their lifetime.[6] Childbirth is the single biggest risk factor for POP, especially if you have experienced a prolonged labour, instrumental delivery, a large baby, a third- or fourth-degree tear (see page 66), or have birthed multiple babies.

While you might not notice any symptoms at the start of your motherhood journey, deep muscle injuries or damage to the connective tissue during birth can slowly weaken the pelvic floor muscles over time, leading to longer-term complications. If any of this resonates with you, please make an appointment with your doctor sooner rather than later to avoid the symptoms becoming worse in later years.

While pregnancy can stretch the tissues and birth can damage them further, it's the lack of early pelvic floor rehab that can make it worse in the long term. If you don't retrain the pelvic floor post-childbirth, the muscles stay weak and lax to a degree. That means they cannot hold up the pelvic organs as well as they could previously and they begin to either shift or bulge down. Even simple things such as laughing, coughing, sneezing, or lifting up your child can put downward pressure on the pelvic organs.

Then, when menopause arrives and oestrogen levels drop, those areas of your body affected by birth, such as your vulva, vagina, and pelvic floor, which may already have scar tissue, nerve sensitivity, or structural weakness, often become more symptomatic:

- Scar tissue becomes more rigid and painful due to thinning vaginal walls, making sex or even smear tests more uncomfortable.
- Prolapse symptoms (such as a bulging feeling or pelvic heaviness) may worsen as the connective tissues lose support.
- Urinary incontinence may become more frequent or severe, especially stress incontinence or urgency.
- Nerve sensitivity from old perineal injuries can be amplified by hormonal changes.

So, while pelvic changes are a natural part of menopause, those who've had traumatic or difficult births often feel the impact more sharply in their 50s and beyond. That's why it's never too late to seek help.

What you can do

- **Speak to your doctor:** There are treatment options available for POPs, including oestrogen preparations and even surgery. You deserve to feel supported and not embarrassed or ignored.
- **See a pelvic health physiotherapist:** They're brilliant at assessing what's going on and can build a plan that works

for your body (see page 73). In the UK, they're available on the NHS.

- **Consider weight management:** You are not alone in this. If you find your weight has become an issue, speak to your doctor who can refer you to weight management services and support you better in losing weight, which will reduce the pressure on your pelvic floor.

'Is My Discharge Normal?'

'Discharge' – it's a funny word isn't it? Vaginal discharge is still a bit of a taboo topic, often whispered about or hidden away. I always note the way women react in my clinic whenever I mention it. For some women, it's just a symptom, but, for many, the word alone evokes a disgusted, sometimes even shameful expression.

Women often feel too embarrassed to speak about vaginal discharge with their doctor for fear of judgement and it makes me sad that we have been raised like this – that something that is so normal has been stigmatized for so long.

So, let's change that. Every woman has discharge. In most cases, it is totally normal, but it can change at different stages of our cycles, hormonal life stages (puberty, pregnancy, childbirth, and menopause), as well as during infections. Learning what is and isn't normal is vital, so let's break it down.

The early mum days

After having a baby, vaginal discharge changes completely, yet it's something many women aren't informed about and that can cause mild panic. Lochia (see page 64) can last for up to six weeks and typically changes from bloody discharge like a period to pinky/brown discharge as things settle, and eventually yellow/creamy coloured discharge. This is all very normal and simply part of the natural healing process. However, if it does not settle down after six weeks or it becomes heavier, smells bad, or is accompanied by pain, you need to get this checked by your health visitor or doctor as it could be a sign of infection.

During breastfeeding, oestrogen levels drop and stay low for that time and this causes more dryness and irritation, known as vaginal atrophy (we'll look at this more closely in Chapter 4 – see page 95). This can increase your risk of vaginal infections by changing the vaginal microbiome, so infections like thrush and bacterial vaginosis (BV) are common (see page 98 for more on these).

After the initial few months postpartum

At this stage, vaginal discharge should settle back to what was normal for you pre-baby – though please bear in mind that this varies from woman to woman, so what is 'normal' for other women may not be for you.

Mid-cycle, normal discharge tends to be clear and stringy (imagine egg whites) and then, just before your period is due, it can look creamy or white. The amount can vary depending on factors like ovulation, stress, or if you work out a lot. I always recommend tracking the cyclical changes in your discharge because once you identify your normal pattern, it's easy to spot a change (see 'What you can do' on the following page).

Your period should return (though this varies from anywhere from two to three months to up to a year postpartum) and, if it doesn't or you find that the kind of discharge you are now having is different, it's always worth getting it checked. Your doctor will take a history, do an examination, and may carry out some swab tests to rule out an infection.

Peri/menopause

Peri/menopause brings with it a whole other wave of change which, in some ways, mimics that first year postpartum as oestrogen starts to fall again. You can experience vaginal dryness, itchiness, soreness, more frequent infections, or foul-smelling discharge, and often women can be misdiagnosed or dismissed as having thrush, BV, or a urinary tract infection (UTI) and treated with antibiotics when the underlying cause may be vaginal atrophy. Don't fall into that trap. If something is happening on repeat, your vagina is trying to communicate with you – and you need to be investigated and managed accordingly.

What you can do

- **Track your changes:** I know many women feel hesitant or embarrassed when talking to their doctor about discharge. Something that can help is to track your changes and write down what you have noticed – including the colour, consistency, smell, texture, and timing. You can then hand this to your doctor without having to go into detail. It's always healthy, even if in a long-term relationship, to have a sexual health screen if you spot any changes.
- **Don't minimize it:** You know your body best, so be its advocate.
- **Ask for a swab:** If infections are recurrent, ask about hormonal factors. It's also worth considering whether it could be perimenopause.

'When Should I Be Worried About Breast Changes?'

As I said at the start of this chapter, even though breast changes are not linked to issues 'down below', it's so important that you know what your 'normal' looks and feels like. Regular self-checking throughout your life – from the teen stage to forever after – means that, if or when there is a new lump or bump, skin change, or pain, you spot it straight away.

Sadly, breast cancer is a genuine risk for women. It is the most commonly diagnosed cancer among women worldwide accounting for approximately 2.3 million new cases in 2022 which represents almost 12 per cent of all new cancer cases globally.[7]

I advise to self-check your breasts once a month at a time outside of your period window (see my tips on page 88).

Postnatal breasts – nobody warns you!

During pregnancy, you feel the changes in your breasts already as they prepare for breastfeeding, but irrespective of how many pregnancies you go through, it still comes as a surprise how quickly they change. This amplifies immediately after the baby arrives and, whether you are breastfeeding or not, oestrogen and progesterone plummet and prolactin surges to stimulate milk production. The result is you can end up with:

- **Engorgement:** Full, tight, sore, and hot breasts.
- **Lumps and bumps:** These are often the result of blocked milk ducts.
- **Asymmetry:** This is very normal but causes a lot of panic.
- **Leakage, swelling, and tenderness on repeat:** Ouch!

Something else I see in mums, especially in the early weeks after birth, is mastitis. This is inflammation of the breast tissue, which is often caused by a blocked milk duct or infection, and usually happens during breastfeeding. Symptoms to look out for include:

- fever
- pain in the breast
- red skin
- heat over the tender part
- hardening of the breast
- feeling generally unwell

If you notice any of these symptoms, there are some things you can do at home to help ease them:

- **Keep feeding or expressing:** Even from the sore side (it helps unblock the duct).
- **Try compresses:** Use warm compresses before feeding and cold compresses after feeding for pain relief.
- **Consider massage:** Gently massage the lump towards the nipple while feeding or when in the shower.
- **Prioritize self-care:** Rest, hydrate, and go braless or wear something non-restrictive. Take paracetamol or ibuprofen to help with any pain and fever.

Please see your doctor if:

- symptoms haven't improved after 24 hours of home treatment
- you develop a high fever
- you feel very unwell
- there's pus or blood coming from the nipple
- you suspect an abscess (a swollen, painful lump that doesn't shift)

Antibiotics may be needed if symptoms don't improve – but, don't worry, you can keep breastfeeding during treatment.

Alongside these postpartum changes, monthly hormonal shifts can also cause:

- pre-period tenderness
- lumpy breasts which settle post-period
- swelling or heaviness

In my clinic, I hear it all – from women delaying coming in because they felt unsure or embarrassed to being afraid of what we might diagnose. Mothers especially, who often put their healthcare needs at the bottom of the pile, will delay seeking help, and what I need to say loud and clear is that early detection of any breast changes should be a priority. Not every lump is cancer, but we have to be able to rule out any worrying changes, and delaying coming in can be a risky move.

Peri/menopausal breast changes

This phase can feel like puberty, albeit now with a mortgage and no sleep. As your oestrogen levels start to fluctuate, your breasts change too. You may notice:

- random soreness
- lumpier breasts
- loss of fatty tissue and less full breasts
- occasional twinges or shooting pains

However, if you notice that something is persisting and new, please get it checked. While breast cancer can occur at any age, we know the risk increases as we get older and, for women, peri/menopause is a crucial time to be extra vigilant.

When to seek help

There are some symptoms that should prompt you to book an appointment with your doctor:

- a new and persisting lump that stays the same, even after feeding
- redness with fever and flu-like symptoms (this could possibly be mastitis)
- any nipple inversion, rashes, change in shape in one breast compared to the other, bleeding, or crusting that is persisting
- skin dimpling or swelling

What you can do

- **Look:** Stand in front of a mirror, with your arms down and then raised. Look for skin or nipple changes, such as dimpling, as well as changes in size, symmetry, and shape.
- **Feel:** Use the flat of your fingers to press down firmly and go round each breast as if it were a clock face, remembering that breast tissue extends into the collarbone and armpit so feel those areas too.
- **Repeat:** Check your breasts regularly (around once a month).

Punam's Prescription

Get comfortable with the new you

Have a look down below! As much as it might seem like the worst suggestion, please do it. You wouldn't hesitate to look at your arm or your leg, so why shy away from looking at and learning more about your genitalia?

With a mirror, have a look – does it look OK to you? Have a feel – does it feel normal? Note any areas of numbness, pain, sensitivity, redness, or deformity. If you have any concerns, see your doctor. I promise you it's nothing to feel weird about – it's important to let your doctor know if you have any concerns so they can pick up any early issues.

Track your bowels and keep a 'water works' diary

Do this for the first few weeks after birth and note down any abnormal symptoms, such as:

- passing blood clots larger than a 50p coin (about 4cm across)
- struggling to pee
- ongoing soreness
- unpleasant vaginal smell
- constipation or sluggish bowels
- leaking poo
- piles (haemorrhoids)

These things are more common than people realize, but that does not mean you have to put up with it. Keeping a diary like this can help to identify problems early. If you are worried, speak to your doctor, nurse, midwife, or health visitor – this diary then makes for an excellent diagnosis tool.

Do your pelvic floor exercises

As a society, we've normalized turning to using lady pads. We've normalized avoiding the things that we enjoy. But we haven't normalized pelvic floor rehabilitation, especially after childbirth. We end up joking about it, crossing our legs when we sneeze, and blaming it on 'mum life'. But so many women miss out on things like playing with their kids, exercising, and even just laughing because they're so scared that they're going to leak. Pads and avoidance are like putting a plaster over the problem. They manage the symptoms to a degree, but they don't treat the underlying cause, whereas getting help to actually strengthen and support the pelvic floor does.

So, I think this is worth repeating as it's so important: practise your pelvic floor exercises from postpartum through to menopause – and beyond! If you can, check with a pelvic health physiotherapist to ensure you are performing them correctly. In the UK, you can request to see one when you are in hospital after the birth, or your health visitor or GP can help refer you.

If you don't have access to a pelvic health physio, there is some useful advice and a 'how to' video on the NHS website (www.nhs.uk), and trusted resources like the NHS-backed Squeezy app can guide you through pelvic floor exercises. Even doing a few minutes of the right exercises consistently can make a big difference.

If you're experiencing bowel incontinence, even if it's just occasional leakage or urgency, this is something a pelvic health physio can help with too.

Schedule in monthly breast checks

Tie self-checks into a date you would never forget like payday. Do it in bed, in the shower, while putting body lotion on – there's no right or wrong time or way; just try stacking it into a routine you already have.

Set a recurring phone alert or reminder in your diary as a non-negotiable meeting with yourself to 'check your boobs' – it only takes two minutes, but it can be life-saving.

Final Thoughts

If you've ever thought that 'something isn't right down there', you're not alone – and you're not imagining it either. We don't talk enough about what really happens to our bodies after birth, not just in the early days, but years, or even decades later. From pelvic floor weakness to incontinence, prolapse, painful sex, and unresolved trauma, too many women are left to cope alone, thinking it's 'just what happens' after motherhood. But none of this is inevitable. And none of it should be dismissed.

Our bodies are incredibly resilient, but they also carry stories: of childbirth, recovery, sacrifice, and survival. Perimenopause often brings these stories to the surface, revealing symptoms that have been bubbling under for years. This isn't ageing, it's the long-term impact of birth catching up, and it deserves care, not silence.

So, if you're leaking, aching, dreading sex, your breasts have changed, or you feel like something's just not quite right, speak up. Track your symptoms. Ask for help. Push for answers because you deserve to feel well, strong, and supported. There is help available if you need it – not just in the postpartum period, but in every chapter of your motherhood journey.

CHAPTER 4

'I'll Never Have Sex Again ... Or Will I?'

REGAINING SEXUAL DESIRE THROUGH THE DECADES

We explored problems 'down below' in the last chapter, but now it's time to focus on sex. Let's start by saying it as it is: sex after having a baby is just different. Having a child can significantly change the way you feel, think about, and experience sex – and this can persist throughout a woman's lifetime. It is one of the most common things women whisper to me during their postnatal visits and, indeed, what my mum friends chat about a lot!

Most women at their six-week postnatal visit will be asked to consider different contraception options. If I had a pound for every time a woman has said to me, 'No thanks, the birth was the best contraception' or 'Abstinence – I'm never going through that again', honestly, I'd be a millionaire by now. Sadly, though, for many women, abstinence becomes a reality, not out of choice, but because of the damage or complications they experienced during birth.

If you have ever wondered why sex has changed, why you've lost your sex drive, why you're more prone to UTIs, or how your hormones are evolving, then this is your must-read chapter. My intention is not to overwhelm you, but to empower you with facts and compassion. It's time to end the silence and shame around talking about libido and offer you the help and support you need.

> ## When to seek help
>
> If you're suffering from any of the symptoms below, please reach out to your family doctor as soon as possible:
>
> - feeling dry down below, especially when having sex
> - a burning sensation
> - pain during sex
> - a persistent sense of rawness down there
> - recurrent UTIs
> - heaviness or pressure sensation in the vagina

'It's Sore When I Have Sex'

I hear this in clinic from so many mothers, and studies show that pain during sex (known in the medical world as 'dyspareunia') is common after childbirth, with research indicating that around one-third of women report pain with intercourse in the months following birth, yet many think they simply have to live with it rather than seek help.[1] Well, I'm here to tell you that you don't.

It's important to understand that there are lots of physiological changes post-birth that can make sex uncomfortable or even painful after having a baby. Let's take a look at some of the most common causes I see in my clinic.

Vaginismus

For some women, painful sex is caused by a condition called vaginismus. This is when the vaginal muscles involuntarily spasm and tighten in response to either a gynaecological examination (smear) or intercourse. Vaginismus can cause serious issues, not just with intimacy but also with avoiding essential life-saving screening tests and examinations (see page 30 for more on managing that first smear test after birth).

Vaginal infections, such as thrush, can lead to vaginismus, though the reasons behind vaginismus aren't always so obvious and the root cause is often trauma – feeling anxious or fearful about sex; having an instrumental birth or suffering deep tears; having had a painful or distressing sexual experience; or going through a difficult medical exam. If this sounds like you, it's important you know there is help out there in the form of specialist psychologists. When left unaddressed, these physical and psychological patterns can become embedded, so it is important to seek help early.

Treatment can vary from therapy and relaxation techniques to pelvic floor exercises and vaginal trainers (devices used to gently stretch the vagina). Please know that you're not alone and there is support out there.

Hormonal shifts

Another cause for pain during intercourse is changing hormones. After birth, oestrogen levels drop sharply and, for many women, this leads to vaginal dryness, sensitivity, and discomfort, especially during sex. If you're breastfeeding, these oestrogen levels can stay low for much longer, because breastfeeding keeps another hormone, prolactin, high, and prolactin naturally suppresses oestrogen production. So, when do things return to normal? It really depends on whether and how long you're breastfeeding for, and how your body individually responds. In women who aren't breastfeeding, oestrogen usually begins to rebound within the first six to eight weeks after birth. But in those who are exclusively breastfeeding, oestrogen can remain low for many months, sometimes until breastfeeding stops or reduces significantly.

It's important to say that this drop in oestrogen is normal, and we also experience it later in life during peri/menopause, but it can cause the vaginal walls to become drier, thinner, and less elastic than they were pre-pregnancy. This condition is called vaginal atrophy, or atrophic vaginitis. Thankfully, more awareness of this condition has been raised in recent years, but more as something that happens during the perimenopause and menopause – rarely is it acknowledged in the context of the postpartum period, when many women struggle with vaginal irritation, dryness, discomfort, or pain during intercourse. Please don't suffer in silence and speak to your doctor about the options outlined on page 101.

Perineal tears

Scar tissue from a perineal tear doesn't just vanish after birth, but it evolves with you. In the early postnatal weeks, it can feel sore, tight, or even sensitive. Over time, however, it should settle, but breastfeeding, hormonal shifts, or even sex can trigger discomfort. There are things that can help if this is you, such as seeing a pelvic health physiotherapist (see page 73), using topical oestrogen (see 'What you can do' on page 101), or scar massaging.

'But I had a C-section, why do I still find sex so painful?'

I get asked this sometimes because many women presume that a vaginal birth would be the cause for sex feeling different. However, sex is dependent on lots of different variables and, when you have a C-section, you will still experience the same fluctuation in hormones, you are still susceptible to birth trauma, and your body still undergoes a huge shake-up – regardless of the way you birthed your baby.

Pelvic floor dysfunction

This is one of the most common, yet most under-recognized, causes of pain during sex after childbirth. It refers to any problem with the strength, tone, or coordination of the pelvic floor muscles, which support the bladder, bowel, and reproductive organs.

What the science says

After pregnancy and birth, especially if there was a long labour, a forceps delivery, or tearing, these muscles can become weakened, overstretched, or overly tight. And here's the surprising bit: some women don't just have weakness, they have tension, where the muscles are constantly clenched without them even realizing. This imbalance can lead to:

- pain with penetration or deep discomfort during sex
- burning or stinging sensations
- a feeling of tightness or 'blockage'
- ongoing bladder or bowel issues (like urgency, leaking, or incomplete emptying)

It's not just physical either – stress, trauma (including birth trauma), and anxiety can all cause the pelvic floor to hold tension, much like how we clench our jaw or shoulders without realizing it.

The good news is that pelvic floor dysfunction is very treatable. A pelvic health physiotherapist (see page 73) can assess your muscle tone and teach you how to relax or strengthen the muscles appropriately because it's not just about doing more Kegels, it's about doing the right ones in the right way for *your* body.

Recurrent urinary tract infections

As we have already seen, oestrogen is responsible for A LOT! When it drops, it also impacts the lining of the urethra (where you pee from) making it more fragile. Without oestrogen support, the tissues stay fragile and vulnerable, hence why some women find that while antibiotics clear UTIs in the moment, the problem keeps coming back.

The vagina also has its own community of microscopic bacteria and organisms whose job it is to help protect the vagina and keep things in balance, like the gut microbiome. Many women still do not know about or understand how important the vaginal microbiome is, but it's vital to look after it, especially during pregnancy and beyond when fluctuating hormones truly start to impact it. A healthy vaginal microbiome keeps the vagina slightly acidic with a pH between 3.8 and 4.5. However, things like hormonal changes, antibiotics, douching (see box below) or using scented washes, sex, stress, poor sleep, and even tight synthetic underwear can all throw it off.

After childbirth, with the drop in oestrogen, the vaginal walls become thin, which means the number of good bacteria also reduces. The pH rises which leaves you more prone to infections like UTIs, thrush (candida), and BV. I've listed the most common symptoms of these infections in the box below as they are quite different. If anything feels 'off' to you, please see your doctor as soon as possible.

Is it a UTI, thrush, or BV?
Here's how to tell the difference:

UTI symptoms
- burning or stinging when you pee
- needing to go urgently or more often than usual
- lower tummy pain or pressure
- cloudy or strong-smelling pee
- occasionally, fever or feeling shaky if it spreads

Thrush (candida) symptoms
- thick, white discharge (like cottage cheese)
- intense itching or burning around the vulva
- redness, swelling, or soreness
- pain during sex or when peeing

BV symptoms
- thin, greyish-white discharge
- strong fishy smell (often worse after sex)
- usually no itching or soreness
- not sexually transmitted, but can be triggered by a pH imbalance (for example, douching, a new partner, or using scented products)

Some simple things you can do to help support your vaginal microbiome post-birth include:

- **Avoiding harsh soaps and chemicals when washing:** Instead, wash with simple warm water or use unscented soap.
- **Wearing breathable cotton underwear:** This is especially important in the first few weeks and months post-childbirth.
- **Keeping yourself hydrated:** Water helps to flush out the bacteria.
- **Using vaginal moisturizers/probiotics:** There is evidence to show that these can help restore the vaginal pH and can also keep the tissues supple.[2]
- **Limiting unnecessary antibiotics:** Antibiotics absolutely have a place in treating certain infections. However, to reduce antibiotic resistance and protect the vaginal microbiome, it's important to limit them when they are not

necessary. Please act on the advice of your doctor and don't stop taking any prescribed antibiotics without medical guidance and support.

If you are getting repeated UTIs postnatally, do not dismiss it and suffer in silence. You need to track your symptoms, see your doctor, and ask them to investigate whether there may be an underlying hormonal imbalance that could be making you more susceptible.

The truth about douching

Douching means washing out the inside of your vagina with water, often using a spray, bottle, or a specially marketed product. There are hundreds of them on the shelves and I get why women feel confused. Some women douche because they want to feel clean, especially after sex or during their period – but here's the truth: your vagina doesn't need cleaning on the inside. It actually self-cleans, which many women don't know.

Douching also disrupts the natural balance of the healthy bacteria in your vaginal microbiome, raises your pH, and makes you more likely to get infections like thrush, BV, and even pelvic inflammatory disease (PID). It can also increase your risk of fertility problems if used long term.

So, despite all the marketing, I strongly advise you to skip the sprays and 'feminine washes', even if the packaging says 'pH balanced'. Wear cotton underwear and have a quick rinse with warm water on the outside only (the vulva) – your vagina will thank you.

When sex is painful in later life

While much of this chapter so far has been centred around the postpartum era, for some women, sexual discomfort can persist well into perimenopause and beyond. That's because unresolved issues like scar tissue, pelvic floor dysfunction, or untreated pain can carry on silently for years, only to resurface or worsen when hormones shift again later in life. As oestrogen levels drop and vaginal tissue becomes thinner and less stretchy, it can make any scar tissue feel tighter and possibly sore again, especially during intercourse. Even decades later, old scars can feel tender, rigid, or prone to itching and splitting.

If sex is still uncomfortable years after birth, it's worth getting assessed, especially by a pelvic health physiotherapist, family doctor, or women's health specialist. Topical oestrogen (see below) and scar massage can also help.

Although these symptoms all sound physical, sadly they spill into other areas of a woman's life too, such as confidence and self-esteem, which is hard when you have just undergone the major life event that is childbirth or are going through peri/menopause. If you are affected by uncomfortable or painful sex, whether it's six months or sixteen years after birth, don't ignore it. Your pelvic floor might be trying to tell you something.

What you can do

- **Don't just put up with it:** While it's common for sex to feel uncomfortable or painful after birth, it's not normal. Please speak to your doctor or a pelvic health physiotherapist – there is support and help available, but you need to reach out first. Your doctor will help to determine the root cause of the issue – is it an infection, a poorly healed wound, scar tissue, vaginal dryness? – and treatment can then be tailored to that.

- **Use vaginal moisturizers and lubricants:** These have been shown to work so don't feel embarrassed if you need to use them.

- **Try topical oestrogen:** You don't need to be perimenopausal to benefit from vaginal oestrogen. After childbirth, particularly if you're breastfeeding, oestrogen levels can remain low for months and this can cause the vaginal tissues to become thin, dry, and more sensitive, leading to discomfort, especially during sex or around healing scars. Topical (local) oestrogen, such as creams, pessaries, or vaginal tablets, can safely be used to restore moisture and elasticity in the vaginal tissues, support healing, and improve comfort. It has very low absorption into the bloodstream, is considered safe during breastfeeding under a doctor's guidance, and does not carry the same risks as systemic hormone therapy. It's a simple but often underused option and one that can make a significant difference to postpartum recovery and well-being.

'I'm Just Not in the Mood'

In clinic, women say things to me like, 'I just can't be bothered with sex anymore', 'I don't feel like myself', and 'I'm not sure what's wrong with me' all the time. If this is you, please stop beating yourself up – low libido after birth, and beyond, is actually very common and there are several reasons why it happens.

Firstly, your hormones are all over the shop. Though you may find that your libido picks up around the time of ovulation as oestrogen levels peak, as oestrogen and testosterone levels start to fall at other times in your cycle or in peri/menopause, many women notice that they feel flat, disconnected, and less interested in sex.

Then there's vaginal atrophy (the thinning of the vaginal tissues we discussed earlier), which can cause dryness, tightness, and discomfort, which, understandably, makes intimacy feel unappealing and even painful sometimes. You might also have stitches or be feeling the baby blues or have anxiety and low mood (more on this in Chapter 7), and therefore you simply won't feel like having sex. Psychological symptoms such as fear, trauma, or shame also play their part and can have a big impact on your libido.

Low libido isn't just about hormones or physiological issues though; it's often your body's way of saying, 'I'm overwhelmed, I need a break', which brings us back to the mental overload or exhaustion that comes with motherhood that we explored in Chapter 2. Many mums are constantly thinking for everybody else – they're managing work, home, family, and everything in between. Your cup is full or over-spilling, and there's just no space for desire when your brain never switches off.

What the science says

Some researchers have explored how stress and the emotional load affect female desire. Studies show that, for many women, especially those juggling work, parenting, and care responsibilities, stress acts like a brake on libido. In her book, *Come as You Are*, educator and researcher Dr Emily Nagoski describes this through the idea of desire being responsive rather than spontaneous – that is, our brains need to feel safe, calm, and connected for the body to follow.[3] In the context of motherhood, when your brain is constantly on, it makes sense that intimacy can feel far from reach. It's not in your head – it's in your nervous system, your hormones, your muscles, and your lived reality as a mother doing a lot, with very little rest.

You might also simply feel 'touched out' – when you are needed all day in a caring capacity, the last thing you want at the end of the day is more touch and intimacy. I remember one of my friends saying to me once that, by the end of every day, this is how she felt. I hadn't had kids at this point and didn't fully understand it and she explained that she just didn't want to be near anyone and needed her own space after her three-year-old went to sleep. This was causing issues in her marriage as she couldn't face even cuddling her partner because all day her toddler needed her for cuddles, attention, touching, playing, co-sleeping – you name it. After I had my own kids, I fully understood what she meant. Even the toilet becomes a communal space when you have little ones – and, after a while, this is draining and can have an impact on how open you feel to intimacy with your partner.

Many women also struggle with body confidence after having a baby, whether it's changes to their weight, scars, stretch marks, or simply not feeling like themselves anymore, and this can make you feel self-conscious during sex. It takes time to reconnect with your body after it's been through so much. Be kind to it, and to yourself. Intimacy isn't just physical, it's also emotional, and it begins with feeling safe, seen, and accepted in the skin you're in.

Now, I don't want it to seem like I am suggesting that men don't feel the emotions and challenges that new parenthood brings, but they don't have the same physiological experiences and so don't always understand why women change as much as they do during that postpartum period and beyond, which is why it's so important to talk about this more. I know a lot of women feel really uncomfortable bringing up sex drive, but please don't be embarrassed. We need to end this stigma and, with honest communication, compassion, shared responsibilities, and medical support, things absolutely can improve because you deserve to feel like you again (see page 108 for my tips on what you can do).

One mum in her late 30s came to see me after her second child. She said, 'It's like I've just switched off. I don't feel like me, I don't even recognize myself in the mirror, and the thought of sex feels like one more job I'm failing at.' She wasn't distressed, just flat and burnt out. She loved her partner and there were no relationship issues, but she felt completely disconnected from her body. Between broken sleep, nursery drop-offs, work deadlines, and the endless mental juggling act, desire simply hadn't crossed her mind in months. What she needed wasn't just hormone checks, it was space, support, and reconnection with herself. We talked about the nervous system, stress, and the role of safety and slowness in desire. She agreed to having some cognitive behavioural therapy (CBT) and opened up to her partner more about it, and, with time, she started to feel like herself again – not by forcing sex, but by learning to prioritize her own needs for the first time in years.

When desire disappears in later life

Loss of libido is difficult during the peri/menopause era, particularly as we have been through the years of juggling the demands of motherhood, work, and life, and just when we think, 'Maybe now it'll ease off', we are struck down by our hormones. It's just not fair!

Hormonal shifts are, once again, the driving factors for loss of libido. As we've seen, as oestrogen drops, it can lead to vaginal atrophy, which means you will lack lubrication down below and therefore not feel comfortable during intercourse, which is a huge turn-off. Another hormone involved is testosterone – yes, we women produce testosterone too – which also starts to fall and causes a loss of desire. If you speak to your doctor, they can help with replacing these hormones (see also 'What you can do' overleaf).

Fatigue and mental load are also factors that can influence libido in midlife. As we saw in Chapter 2, this stage of life often comes with more demands – perhaps supporting children in their teens/adulthood or looking after ageing relatives alongside work – and, when we are stressed and burnt out, it can affect how we feel towards others.

The bottom line is that you are not frigid and you are not alone: many mothers experience a shift in themselves, in their identity, and in their desire and needs in their 40s and 50s. While life may look different and you may feel like you've changed, it's about embracing the shift and believing that sex can still feel rich, intimate, and fulfilling, but, for this, you need support.

Sadly, due to societal pressures, women often feel guilty when they're not in the mood for sex. You might question your love for your partner and vice versa, but this is where an understanding of the norm is important and open communication is key.

What you can do

- **Be gentle on yourself:** Remember – you are only human! Practise the love and compassion that you give to your family and friends on yourself too.
- **Accept medical help and support:** There are several safe and effective treatments that can be offered to women experiencing low libido. For younger women, especially after childbirth or during breastfeeding, when oestrogen levels are naturally lower, options include vaginal oestrogen for dryness or pain during sex, which is safe to use even if you're breastfeeding or not perimenopausal. Testosterone may also be considered under specialist guidance for women with low sexual desire. For women with menstrual cycle-related symptoms, such as PMS or PMDD, there are treatments ranging from progestogen-only contraception to psychological support or referral to a specialist. Treatment should always be individualized and based on your symptoms, not just your age or life stage. For women in peri/menopause, help may come in the form of HRT, which supports hormone balance and can improve energy, mood, and libido. Testosterone is another option for some women – a carefully monitored dose can really help restore desire. Vaginal oestrogen can also make a huge difference to comfort, confidence, and intimacy, and it is safe and effective. You are not a failure for taking these and it does not have to be forever.

• **Make space for yourself again.** That might mean
  putting in place better boundaries, like saying no to
  social plans when you're exhausted, asking your partner
  to take over bedtime so you can go for a walk, or carving
  out 15 minutes in the morning for some quiet time before
  the day begins. It might mean starting therapy to process
  what you've been through, or having open conversations
  with your partner about how your relationship has
  changed and what you both need now. It might simply
  mean resting: lying down for 10 minutes instead of folding
  laundry, drinking a hot drink before it goes cold, or
  watching a show that's just for you. This is not selfish –
  it is essential.

Punam's Prescription

Ease into sex after birth

If sex is painful or you just don't feel in the mood for intimacy, here are my tips for easing back in:

- **Open up:** Honest communication with your partner is the first and most powerful step in connecting and building trust again. Please don't pretend that everything is all right, or just assume that this is what sex will be like for you now – it's not.
- **Take it slowly:** Try exploring your body by yourself at first and remember that sex doesn't have to mean penetration. Take time to just 'be' with your partner, relax with each other, and take things slowly.
- **Seek help:** As we've discussed throughout this chapter, there is so much help and support out there. Please reach out, whether that's to your doctor, a pelvic health physiotherapist (see page 73), or a counsellor – don't suffer in silence; you are not alone in this.

Consider therapy

If there is any history of trauma, it's worth speaking to a trained professional to help you address any underlying emotional issues that might be impacting on your libido. Please also revisit Chapter 1 for practical advice and support if you have had a traumatic birth.

Choose your contraception

For most women, sex is the last thing on their mind after they have given birth. However, you would be surprised by the number of unplanned pregnancies that come about during those first few weeks and months postpartum, which makes for tricky consultations.

You may have heard that you can't get pregnant while breastfeeding, but that's a myth. It's true that breastfeeding can delay the return of your periods, especially in the early months. That's because a hormone called prolactin, which supports milk production, also suppresses ovulation. But here's the catch: ovulation happens before your period returns, so you can still get pregnant without ever seeing a bleed.

The lactational amenorrhoea method (LAM – using breastfeeding as a contraception method) can offer some protection, but only if you're exclusively breastfeeding, doing so around the clock, your baby is under six months old, and your periods haven't come back. Even then, it's not foolproof.

If you're not ready for another pregnancy, it's worth chatting to your doctor about contraception – ideally before you even leave the hospital. Below is a quick summary of your options.

Immediately (hours/days) after birth
- **Condoms:** These are hormone-free and can be used instantly.
- **Progesterone-only pill:** This is safe while breastfeeding and highly effective.
- **Contraceptive injection (for example, Depo-Provera):** This can be given before being discharged from hospital; again, it is safe if you are breastfeeding.
- **Hormonal or copper coil (IUD/IUS):** This can be inserted within forty-eight hours of birth or delayed to four weeks post-birth.
- **Implant (for example, Nexplanon):** This can be offered before leaving hospital.

From three weeks
- **Combined oral contraceptive pill:** This has oestrogen and progesterone in it, so you cannot take it if you are breastfeeding or have any contraindications (check with your doctor).

From six weeks
- All methods are safe including the coil, implants and, if you wish, sterilization.

If you are breastfeeding
Not all contraceptive methods are equally suitable during breastfeeding, but there are safe and effective options, including:

- **Progestogen-only methods:** These are sometimes called 'mini pills':
  - progestogen-only pill (POP)
  - injectable (Depo-Provera)
  - hormonal IUS (for example, Mirena)
- **Implant:** This is considered safe and does not affect milk supply, even when started soon after birth.
- **Barrier methods:** Condoms, diaphragms, and cervical caps are safe at any time.
- **Non-hormonal methods:** The copper IUD (coil) is safe and effective during breastfeeding, and is typically inserted four weeks postpartum.

Combined hormonal contraceptives (such as the combined pill, patch, or vaginal ring) are not recommended in the first six weeks after birth if you are breastfeeding, due to the potential for oestrogen to reduce milk supply and the increased risk of blood clots in the immediate postpartum period. After six weeks, if breastfeeding is well-established and there are no other medical risk factors, combined hormonal methods can be considered. Always discuss your options with your doctor or contraception provider to find what's best for you.

Final Thoughts

We've seen how motherhood changes your sense of identity as well as your anatomy and physiology. It has an impact on your sleep, your energy levels, your relationships, and, yes, now your vaginal and sexual health too!

I hope you now have a better understanding of the factors that impact sex and intimacy – from overwhelm and body image changes to vaginal dryness, low libido, and possible pelvic trauma. This awareness is the another step to making your health and well-being a priority. Please reach out if you need help – there are so many options available.

CHAPTER 5

'Everything Hurts'

RELIEVING JOINT PAIN AND RECLAIMING YOUR POWER

Almost daily, I hear the same things from mothers in my clinic: 'I don't know what I've done, but my back just isn't the same since I had my baby', 'Everything hurts all the time', or 'I always feel so stiff.' Sometimes, it is days or weeks after their baby was born, and sometimes it is decades later.

These women aren't imagining things. The impact of carrying and delivering your baby can take a significant toll on your musculoskeletal (MSK) system (aka the bones and joints of your body). Your body isn't the same anymore and that's not a flaw, but the result of an incredible physical transformation that leaves no bone, joint, muscle, or ligament untouched.

From the moment you fall pregnant, hormonal shifts and the physical demands of carrying a baby mean that your MSK system begins to adapt. Your pelvis softens. Your spine tilts. Your core stretches. Sadly, unlike elite athletes, new mums rarely get rehab plans or recovery time after giving birth. We are back in action immediately, powered by love, coffee, and survival mode. With that, come the postnatal postural shifts as a result of carrying a baby on your hip, lugging around car seats and changing bags, feeding in awkward positions, standing or rocking for hours, and never really getting enough rest to fully recover! And the impact doesn't end there – years later, as hormone levels drop in peri/

menopause, these earlier MSK changes can resurface or worsen, contributing to joint pain, stiffness, and reduced core strength.

The result of all of this is that a huge number of mums are living for years with stiffness, clicking joints, hip pain, and backache that they quietly accept as part of the job. However, these aren't just signs of wear and tear; they are signs of a system that's been overworked and under-supported – but you don't have to accept them as your 'new normal'.

In this chapter, we will explore why MSK symptoms are so common in mums and how they show up at different stages of motherhood – from newborn life through to the menopause. I'll explain the role hormones play, the long-term effects of not addressing issues early, and the symptoms you should never ignore. More importantly, I'll share practical, evidence-based strategies to help you move better, feel stronger, and reclaim your body, one stretch, lift, and breath at a time.

When to seek help

Most back and joint pain in motherhood is benign, but there are a few warning signs you shouldn't ignore. See your doctor or physiotherapist if you experience:

- pain that wakes you at night and doesn't ease with movement
- pain that is persistent or worsening
- numbness or tingling in your groin, legs, or feet
- new bladder or bowel symptoms, especially loss of control (this could signal cauda equina syndrome, which is a rare but serious medical emergency)
- unexplained weight loss or fever with back pain
- persistent swelling, warmth, or redness in joints
- stiffness that lasts for more than 30 minutes in the morning,

especially if it's symmetrical – this could point to early autoimmune arthritis

It's also worth reaching out if:

- you can't do everyday tasks without discomfort
- you have pelvic heaviness, leaking, or core instability
- you're unsure which movements are safe or helpful
- you suspect peri/menopause or hormonal changes are playing a role

'There's a Gap in My Tummy': The Baby Years

After birth, we expect some bleeding, leaky boobs, and maybe stitches, but what is rarely spoke about is the moment you lie down, lift your head up slightly, and feel a weird dip in the middle of your now wobbly, soft tummy. There's a space, a softness, a gap.

That gap – which affects roughly 60 per cent of women at six weeks postpartum, with around 30 per cent still having it at one year[1] – is known as diastasis recti or divarication. It is a separation of the abdominal muscles that happens in most pregnancies to make space for the growing baby.

So, how do you know you have it? You might notice:

- a bulge or doming when you sit up from lying down
- a gap between your abdominal muscles that you can feel with your fingers
- a sense of weakness in your core or lack of support
- back pain, especially when lifting or standing for long periods
- pelvic floor issues like leaking, heaviness, or prolapse (see Chapter 3)

Very few women are ever checked for diastasis recti or taught to look for it themselves, and most don't even know it's a thing. But here's why it matters: your abdominal wall is a key part of your 'core canister' – along with your diaphragm, pelvic floor, and deep back muscles, these structures work together to manage intra-abdominal pressure, support your spine, and allow you to move efficiently. If one part of that system isn't functioning well – for example, if the abdominal muscles stay separated and weak – then the other parts start to compensate, often leading to overuse, strain, or injury. And guess what usually picks up the slack? Your lower back. That's why so many mums with unresolved diastasis recti complain of persistent backache, pelvic floor dysfunction, or feeling like their core is weak no matter how many crunches they try (which, by the way, can make things worse!).

If diastasis recti doesn't resolve well, over time it can contribute to:

- reduced core strength and stability
- back and pelvic pain
- poor posture or spinal misalignment
- urinary leaking or POP (see Chapter 3)
- a persistent tummy bulge or 'doming'

Diastasis recti is a completely normal adaptation to pregnancy. For most women, the gap naturally begins to close in the first eight weeks after birth, especially as hormone levels settle and the body begins to heal. By around six months postpartum, many women will find the muscles have reconnected to a functional level, but, for others, the separation remains wider or weaker than it should be.

You can do a simple self-check at home:

1. Lie on your back with your knees bent and feet flat on the floor.

2. Place your fingers just above your belly button.
3. Gently lift your head and shoulders slightly off the floor, like starting a crunch, and feel for a gap between the two sides of your abdominal muscles.
4. Measure how many fingers fit into the gap. A gap of more than two finger-widths may indicate diastasis recti.
5. Repeat the check at the belly button, just above it, and just below it. You might also notice a dip, doming, or softness along the midline, which could indicate the tissue is still not providing enough support.

When to seek help

It's worth speaking to your doctor, physiotherapist, or health visitor if:

- the gap doesn't seem to improve over eight to twelve weeks after birth
- you feel your core is weak, unstable, or domes when you lift or move
- you have ongoing back pain, pelvic floor issues, or posture problems
- you're struggling with leaking, heaviness, or bulging in the pelvic area
- you're unsure what's going on and just want a proper check

A women's health physiotherapist can assess your abdominal function and guide you through a safe, tailored recovery plan – often with incredible results. This isn't about 'bouncing back'; healing doesn't have a time limit. It's about rebuilding your foundation, so you feel strong, supported, and able to move without pain.

Symphysis pubis dysfunction

What we don't talk about enough is that pregnancy can also signal the beginning of longer-term joint and connective tissue issues, and something I see a lot in new mums in clinic is symphysis pubis dysfunction (SPD).

A key hormone in pregnancy is relaxin, which plays an important role in preparing your body for birth. It works by softening the ligaments, loosening joints (especially in the pelvis), and allowing the body to stretch and expand as the baby grows. But relaxin doesn't just vanish after birth, it lingers for up to five months, and even longer if you're breastfeeding, which can leave joints feeling wobbly and ligaments looser than usual. That's why conditions like SPD can persist well into your baby's first year – especially if there was trauma during birth or poor postnatal recovery.

The pubic symphysis is the joint at the front of your pelvis. During pregnancy, it widens slightly to accommodate your baby and, sometimes, it doesn't realign well postpartum. Common signs include:

- pain or pressure at the front of the pelvis, inner thighs, or groin
- a 'clicking' or 'shearing' feeling when you walk, climb stairs, or turn over in bed
- pain climbing stairs, lunging, or standing on one leg
- instability in the pelvis or hips when carrying your child

Left untreated, it can become a persistent source of pain – and affect the way you walk, stand, and sit.

SPD is common, but not normal – and it's definitely treatable. A women's health physiotherapist can assess your alignment, muscle imbalances, and pelvic floor, and then build a personalized recovery plan to support your mobility and reduce pain. In the meantime, there are some self-help strategies that can make a difference:

- **Use a pelvic support belt:** This can help stabilize the pelvis and reduce strain when moving around.
- **Keep your legs together:** When getting out of bed, out of the car, or off the sofa, try to move your knees together rather than one at a time to reduce shearing pressure across the pelvis.
- **Sleep with a pillow between your knees:** This helps to keep your hips aligned and reduces strain on the pelvis at night.
- **Avoid heavy lifting and asymmetrical movements:** This is especially important for those that involve twisting or wide steps.
- **Use stairs mindfully:** Take one step at a time or try going up and down sideways if that feels more comfortable.
- **Apply heat or cold packs:** Some women find warmth soothing, while others benefit from cooling inflammation down.
- **Rest regularly and pace yourself:** Listen to your body and don't push through the pain. Break tasks into smaller chunks and build in rest time.

Always flag your symptoms to your midwife, doctor, or physio – early intervention makes a big difference, and you don't have to 'just put up with it'.

Other early postnatal MSK issues

Alongside diastasis recti and SPD, the hormonal changes, mechanical strain, and tissue stretching of pregnancy can unmask or trigger:

- **Pelvic girdle pain (PGP):** Pain around the hips, pelvis, or lower back, often continuing after birth.
- **Sacroiliac joint dysfunction:** Pain where the spine meets the pelvis.

- **Hypermobility spectrum disorders (HSD) or undiagnosed Ehlers-Danlos syndromes:** Sometimes these are first noticed in pregnancy (see box below).
- **Postpartum tendonitis:** Especially in the wrists, thumbs, shoulders, or knees, from lifting and repetitive strain.
- **Early signs of osteoarthritis:** Especially in the hips or knees, which may progress later in life (see page 113 for more on the signs of osteoarthritis).

For some mums, these issues improve with time and support. But for others, this marks the start of a longer MSK journey – one that deserves recognition, rehab, and proper follow-up.

Could it be hypermobility?

Some women, especially those with a long history of joint clicking, muscle fatigue, or 'clumsiness', may have underlying joint hypermobility. It often goes unrecognized in childhood and only becomes problematic with hormonal changes, pregnancies, or after years of overcompensation.

Hypermobility is more common in those who were previously dancers, gymnasts, or 'double-jointed' as kids, and can make your joints more mobile than average, but less stable.

Signs include:

- joints that click, pop, or partially dislocate
- frequent sprains or strains
- being easily injured or fatigued after normal activity
- slower recovery from exercise
- family history of hypermobility or connective tissue disorders
- IBS-like symptoms, dizziness, or anxiety (in more complex syndromes)

Pregnancy often worsens hypermobility symptoms because the hormone relaxin adds even more laxity. Without targeted strengthening, joint support can stay compromised for years.

What you can do

- **Get checked by a women's health physiotherapist:** This is hands down the most valuable investment you can make in your body after birth. A specialist physio can assess your abdominal separation, pelvic floor, and joint alignment, and give you personalized rehab guidance.
- **Start with gentle core rehab:** Crunches and planks are not your friend in these early days. Instead, focus on:
  - diaphragmatic breathing
  - transverse abdominis engagement ('belly hugs')
  - heel slides
  - pelvic tilts
  - glute bridges

  These small, subtle moves help rebuild the foundational strength you need to protect your back and pelvis long term.
- **Practise 'exhale on effort':** Whether you're lifting your baby, standing up, or pushing the buggy, breathe out during the effort. This helps activate your core and reduces intra-abdominal pressure.
- **Move mindfully:** Avoid long periods of sitting or standing in the same position. When carrying your baby, alternate sides regularly, use both hands when lifting the car seat, and try not to twist when lifting. You don't need to be perfect, but a little awareness goes a long way.

'I Feel Stiff All the Time': The Toddler Years

By now, your little one's on the move – and so are you. Constantly! You're crawling on the floor, bending to tie tiny shoes, lifting them into car seats, hoisting scooters out of the car boot, and contorting yourself into small spaces at soft play. It's the phase of motherhood when your body gets used (and often abused) in the same repetitive, inefficient ways – day in, day out. No wonder everything starts to feel a bit … stiff and stuck.

Mums at this stage often tell me they're not in pain but feel 'tight' in their bodies – we're talking about those groans when you get off the sofa, those clicks in your neck when you turn your head, and those warning twinges in your lower back when you lean over the bath. I've been there too and it's not fun!

We all tend to question whether it's age catching up with us when it's actually not. It's patterned strain, which means the body has been moving in the same limited, often awkward ways (like carrying a toddler on one hip, leaning over cots, or crouching on the floor) over and over again. Over time, this creates stiffness, muscle imbalances, and tension that can show up as those clicks, twinges, and tightness.

This postural dysfunction is linked with a higher risk of chronic lower back pain – especially in postpartum women.[2] Simple tweaks, however, can make a big difference:

- alternate the hip you carry your child on
- use a backpack or cross-body bag to reduce one-sided strain
- squat or lunge to lift, rather than bending from the waist
- sit upright with support during feeds or screen time

Something I recommend in clinic is to ask someone to take a side-on photo of you in a natural standing position. Look at your head, shoulders, pelvis, and knees. Are you leaning forward? Are your shoulders rounded? Are your hips tilted? Awareness is the first step towards better movement habits.

Mechanical back pain

This is by far the most common diagnosis I see in mums during the toddler years. It's called 'mechanical' because it's caused by how your body moves – or doesn't move – rather than inflammation, arthritis, or nerve damage. It often stems from:

- poor posture (carrying kids on one hip, bending with a curved spine)
- muscle imbalances (underactive glutes, tight hip flexors, weak core)
- lack of movement variety (same chores, same movements, every day)
- injury or just sheer exhaustion

You might feel:

- a dull ache in the lower back, especially by the end of the day
- stiffness when getting out of bed or off the floor
- sharp twinges when you twist, bend, or lift
- relief with gentle movement, heat, or stretching

While it's not dangerous, it's not something to ignore either. Mechanical back pain left unaddressed can snowball into chronic issues, such as persistent lower back pain, sciatica, nerve irritation, postural changes, pelvic instability, or even reduced mobility over time. It can also contribute to tension headaches and impact your sleep, energy levels, and overall quality of life.

What you can do

- **Try 'movement snacks':** You don't need an hour-long class – just two to three minutes of gentle stretching or mobility here and there through the day. Try:
  - cat-cow spinal rolls
  - child's pose
  - pelvic tilts
  - glute bridges
  - wall angels to open tight chest muscles

  I do these while I'm waiting for the kettle to boil, during my lunch break, and while I'm watching the telly or on the phone – we mums are the best at multitasking so we may as well extend it to our health goals!

- **Strengthen your bum:** Your glutes are your pelvic stabilizers – and motherhood often makes them lazy, so we need to wake them up. Some easy ways are:
  - side-lying clamshells
  - glute bridges
  - mini squats
  - resistance band walks

- **Prioritize recovery:** I am realistic and know it isn't always easy to get the seven to nine hours' sleep a night that's recommended, but can you:
  - Nap if your child naps?
  - Use a hot water bottle on stiff areas?
  - Stretch for 5 minutes before bed?

  Small habits, repeated daily, bring big shifts.

'My Joints Are Clicking': Perimenopause

You're past the buggy years, your child is more independent, you're sleeping a bit more (hopefully), you're lifting less, and you're spending less time in awkward toddler-wrangling positions, so why do your joints feel worse? You crouch down to zip up your little one's coat and your knees click. You stretch in bed and your shoulders crack. You go for a jog and feel like the Tin Man. The aches are quieter, but they're there – and they're persistent.

You might brush it off as getting older, but, for many women – especially mothers – this stage marks the beginning of a new hormonal shift: perimenopause. And if you've had children, you may notice that old aches and twinges you thought had gone away suddenly start to creep back in. That's because the physical impact of pregnancy and birth doesn't just disappear – and when oestrogen levels start to dip, the tissues and joints that were already under strain can become more vulnerable. If you had pelvic pain, diastasis recti, or back problems during or after pregnancy that weren't fully addressed, this is often the time they resurface. The result? Stiffness, joint clicks, and that sense that your body just isn't moving like it used to. It's not just perimenopause, it's the long shadow of motherhood showing up in a new season.

When to seek help

Things to watch for in this phase include:

- prolonged morning stiffness
- swollen or red joints
- fatigue that's affecting daily life
- multiple joint pain without clear injury
- symptoms that are symmetrical (like in both hands or knees)
- family history of autoimmune disease
- numbness, tingling, or weakness in limbs

These could be signs of rheumatoid arthritis or another autoimmune condition, which are more common in women in their 30s and 40s than people realize. Often pregnancy is the trigger for onset. You may need:

- blood tests
- referral to rheumatology
- imaging (X-rays, ultrasound, or MRI if indicated)

You're not being dramatic. If it's affecting your quality of life, it's worth investigating.

Let's look more deeply at what's going on during perimenopause when it comes to MSK health.

Oestrogen and joint health

Oestrogen isn't just about periods and hot flushes – it plays a big role in the elasticity of your ligaments and tendons, joint lubrication, collagen production, muscle strength, and inflammation control too. As levels begin to fluctuate – often from your late 30s into your 40s – joints may feel less cushioned, and more brittle or inflamed. Collagen declines too – meaning your soft tissues (like cartilage and fascia – the thin layer of connective tissue that wraps around and supports your muscles, bones, and organs) aren't as springy or well-lubricated as before.

You may notice:

- clicking, cracking, or stiffness in your joints, especially in the mornings
- generalized aches in your neck, shoulders, hips, or fingers
- a sense of 'tightness' or soreness that doesn't go away with rest

- increased injuries and slower healing
- greater sensitivity to repetitive strain
- fatigue, poor sleep, and brain fog alongside these physical symptoms

These can be early signs of perimenopause.

The role of sleep deprivation

Stiffness isn't just about what you do – it's also about what you don't do. And most mums don't sleep enough to allow for proper muscle recovery. When you're carrying the mother load – physically, mentally, and emotionally – that stress and exhaustion don't just stay in your head. They settle into your body too, tightening muscles, reducing flexibility, and leaving you feeling heavier, achier, and more sluggish over time.

As discussed in Chapter 2, chronic sleep deprivation reduces the growth hormone, increases cortisol (your stress hormone), and actually makes your pain threshold lower. That's why everything hurts more when you're tired. It's not just in your head – it's neurochemical.

If anything in this section has resonated with you, you'll be pleased to hear that you can combat the hormonal shifts of perimenopause, preserve muscle strength, and support your joints – and it all comes down to strength training.

Strength training: The key to reclaiming your power

From our mid-30s, we start to lose around 1 per cent of muscle mass per year – a process called 'sarcopenia'. Add oestrogen decline and sedentary work or childcare patterns, and your joints are doing a whole lot more without adequate muscle backup, and so strengthening muscles around the joints (especially the glutes, hamstrings, core, and shoulders) is the single best thing you can do to reduce pain, prevent injury, and build long-term resilience.

This is the stage when strength training isn't just a nice-to-have, it's necessary, and, for decades, women have not been educated about its importance. Strength training is the most effective way to:

- support and stabilize joints
- improve balance and reduce falls
- reduce the risk of osteoporosis
- reduce joint pain

The Royal Osteoporosis Society recommends strength and balance training for all women over the age of 40, especially as they approach menopause.[3]

Here are some simple ways to build your strength:

- **Do bodyweight exercises:** Try squats, lunges, or push-ups against the wall.
- **Use resistance bands:** These are perfect for home workouts.
- **Try hand weights:** They don't have to be heavy; you can even use filled water bottles to start.
- **Focus on form, not load:** Strength training is about quality over quantity.

If you're new to strength work, try free NHS online classes or community classes run by qualified instructors.

One of my patients, a 35-year-old mum of two, told me recently, 'I finally have time to exercise again now the kids are older, but every time I go for a run, my hips seize up the next day. I feel stiffer than I did when I was postpartum!' She'd put it down to age or needing new trainers, but the real culprit was hormonal. We talked through a few options, from gentle strength work to anti-inflammatory nutrition. With a few lifestyle changes and support, she felt more in control of her body again and reassured that she wasn't just 'getting old'. Her story shows us that it's never too late to rebuild strength and feel more supported in your body.

What you can do

- **Address hormonal shifts:**
  If joint pain is accompanied by:
  - mood swings
  - poor sleep
  - hot flushes
  - brain fog
  - irregular cycles
  … then perimenopause may be a contributing factor.
  Speak to your family doctor about:
  - HRT (which can improve joint pain in many women)
  - blood tests (although clinical diagnosis is key in women over 45 as hormones fluctuate so much)
  - bone density scans if at risk of osteoporosis
- **Keep moving (but vary the movement):** Sitting all day = stiffness. But overdoing it in bursts can flare things too. The sweet spot? Frequent, low-impact movement, such as:
  - walking
  - swimming
  - Pilates
  - mobility-focused yoga
  - mini stretching sessions during screen time or work breaks
  Aim for 150 minutes of moderate activity per week, plus two sessions of muscle-strengthening work.
- **Eat to support your joints:** Think:
  - omega-3 fatty acids (found in oily fish, walnuts, and flaxseeds) to help reduce inflammation
  - anti-inflammatory foods such as colourful veg, turmeric, or ginger
  - colourful fruit and veg for antioxidants and joint support

- ○ vitamin D and calcium to support bone health (especially post-40)
- ○ reducing ultra-processed foods and sugar, which can increase inflammation
- ○ Collagen supplements may help some women with joint symptoms, though research on this is mixed.

'Everything Feels Heavy': Menopause

By the time you reach your late 40s or 50s, you've probably stopped carrying babies and wrestling toddlers. You may even have teens now – and yet, you find yourself groaning when you get up from the sofa, struggling to bend and pick things up, and waking up with that deep, dull ache across your lower back. Not sharp, not injury-related – just a constant background presence.

You're not imagining it. For many women, back and joint pain intensify around menopause. And it's not just age – it's oestrogen decline, collagen loss, muscle decline, and often bone changes too. Let's break this down.

Collagen loss

We've covered the importance of oestrogen for joint health in the perimenopause section above. It also plays a major role in collagen production – which is essential for supple muscles and healthy skin. As oestrogen levels drop after menopause, collagen declines by around 30 per cent in the first 5 years.[4] This means stiffer joints, less spring in your step, and slower healing.

Sarcopenia (muscle loss)

As mentioned above, from the age of 40, we naturally lose up to 1 per cent of muscle mass per year – and it accelerates after menopause unless we actively resist it. Less muscle means less support for your spine and joints, leading to that 'everything feels heavy' feeling.

Bone density decline

Oestrogen plays a vital role in keeping your bones strong and healthy, too, by regulating the natural process of bone turnover, where old bone is broken down and new bone is formed. But after menopause, as oestrogen levels drop, bone breakdown begins to outpace bone formation. Over time, this can lead to osteopenia (a lower-than-normal bone density) and, in some women, progress to osteoporosis (a condition where bones become fragile and more prone to fractures).

In the early stages, both osteopenia and osteoporosis are often silent; many women don't realize their bone density is declining until a scan picks it up or they suffer a break after a minor fall. The most common fracture sites are the spine, hips, and wrists.

Some symptoms to watch out for include:

- loss of height over time
- a stooped posture
- back pain from tiny spinal fractures (known as compression fractures)
- fractures after minimal trauma, like tripping or lifting

A simple test called a DEXA scan can check your bone density and help assess your risk – it's quick, painless, and uses low-dose X-rays to measure bone strength. If you've had an early menopause, a family history of osteoporosis, or other risk factors, it's worth discussing this with your doctor.

One in two women over 50 will experience an osteoporosis-related fracture in their lifetime.[5] We can do a lot to try reduce this risk and prevent these fractures as best we can (see 'What you can do' on page 134).

Is it wear and tear or inflammation?

That's the question many women are left asking when the aches and pains start creeping in during their 40s. One minute it's a deep, nagging lower backache. The next, it's a tightness in the hips that just won't shift, or a stiffness in the morning that makes getting out of bed feel like you've aged 20 years overnight. You might even feel the pain radiating around your pelvis, into your thighs, or down your legs like a dull, dragging discomfort that seems to come and go without clear cause.

Sometimes the pain feels muscular or joint-related – what we medics call 'mechanical pain'; it comes from the way your joints, muscles, or posture are working (or not working). This kind of pain is often linked to movement or load, like an ache in your lower back after lifting or a knee twinge when crouching. Other times, the pain feels more inflammatory; it's deeper, more widespread, harder to pinpoint, and often worse in the mornings or after rest. It can feel like your whole body is aching for no obvious reason. For many mums in menopause, it's a combination of both: mechanical strain from years of carrying, bending, and lifting, layered with hormonal changes that increase sensitivity and reduce the body's ability to recover as quickly. Here's how to tell the difference:

Wear and tear (osteoarthritis)	Inflammatory joint pain (autoimmune)
Comes on gradually	Can appear suddenly
Worse after activity	Worse in the morning and gets better as the day goes on
May affect one or two joints (common in hips, knees, and hands)	Often affects multiple joints symmetrically (fingers, wrists)
Feels like stiffness or grinding	Joints feel hot, swollen, or burning
Improves with rest	Improves with movement
No whole-body (systemic) symptoms	Symptoms include fatigue, low-grade fevers, or weight loss

Many women in this phase say to me, 'I just don't feel like myself anymore' and it's no wonder when we layer fatigue, disrupted sleep, hormonal fluctuations, and the emotional load many women are carrying on top of MSK symptoms.

The key is recognizing it early, understanding where it's coming from, and knowing that there is help and support available. You don't have to just put up with it.

When to seek help

Always speak to your doctor if:

- you've had a fall, or notice a height loss of >2cm
- you have persistent or worsening back pain
- you experience new-onset incontinence or bowel changes

- you experience numbness, tingling, or muscle weakness
- you feel exhausted, down, or not yourself for more than a few weeks

You may benefit from:

- blood tests (to check vitamin D, thyroid, and inflammatory markers)
- a DEXA (bone density) scan
- a physio referral or joint injections
- HRT or other hormone-based treatments
- a referral to rheumatology or pain services

What you can do

- **Eat to support your bones:** Key nutrients in menopause include:
  - calcium (700–1,000mg/day from diet and supplements if needed)
  - vitamin D (especially October to March in the UK)
  - protein to maintain muscle mass
  - magnesium, zinc, and vitamin K2 to support bone and joint health
- **Keep moving:** Try:
  - weight-bearing exercise (such as walking, dancing, or stair climbing)
  - resistance training two to three times per week (with bands, weights, or bodyweight)
  - balance training (to prevent falls and improve coordination)

Remember, bone is a living tissue. The more stress you apply to it safely, the stronger it becomes.

- **Stretch smart, strengthen smarter:** Menopausal women often say to me: 'I just need to stretch more.' But often, the real need is strength, so try:
  - short daily mobility: think cat-cow, spinal rolls, or shoulder shrugs
  - isometric holds: like a wall sit or glute bridge
  - Pilates, yoga, or strength circuits adapted for your level
  - guided online classes (see the NHS links on page 128)

  See a physio or personal trainer if you're unsure where to start.
- **Address sleep, stress, and recovery:** As we've seen, poor sleep increases pain perception and stress raises cortisol, which contributes to inflammation and fatigue. In the menopause years, rest becomes just as important as movement.
  - Prioritize sleep hygiene: Even if sleep is broken, protect your wind-down routine.
  - Eat magnesium-rich foods (or supplements).
  - Use heat packs or baths with Epsom salt to ease stiffness.
  - Try gentle yoga or massage.
  - Stay hydrated and nourished: Under-fuelled bodies feel more pain.
  - Consider CBT techniques if pain and sleep anxiety feed each other.
- **Consider HRT:** If there are no contraindications to this for you, HRT can help relieve:
  - joint pain
  - back pain
  - muscle stiffness
  - bone loss
  - sleep disruption (which worsens pain perception)

A 2021 NICE guideline review highlighted that HRT can improve quality of life and MSK symptoms in many menopausal women – especially when started under the age of 60 or within 10 years of menopause.[6] Speak to your doctor if joint pain is affecting your daily life. You don't need to suffer in silence or 'wait it out'.

Punam's Prescription

Do a body audit

Take 5 quiet minutes and ask yourself:

- Do I wake up stiff? Where is the stiffness?
- Do I get sore after sitting, lifting, or walking?
- Can I squat or bend comfortably?
- Do my joints feel stable or do they feel like they're 'catching' or 'giving way'?
- Do I feel connected to my core or do I brace or strain to lift?
- Do I feel stronger than I did a year ago or more fragile?

Awareness is step one. From there, you can start rebuilding.

Track your symptoms

Keep a joint pain diary for a few weeks and note:

- when the pain happens
- which joints are involved
- any accompanying symptoms (fatigue, swelling, and so on)
- your sleep, period cycles, and stress levels

This helps you and your doctor to spot patterns and decide if hormones, autoimmune investigations, or physio might help.

Try the 10/10/10 rule

This simple daily structure is helpful for busy mums who have no time, but want to feel more mobile and in control of their body. It is tried and tested by yours truly.

Commit to 10 minutes of stretching or mobility:

- cat-cow spinal rolls
- child's pose
- supine twists
- pelvic tilts
- shoulder rolls and neck circles

Do 10 bodyweight strength reps:

- squats (or sit-to-stand from a chair)
- glute bridges
- wall push-ups
- standing calf raises
- bird-dogs (for core and back control)

Spend 10 seconds checking your posture (3 times per day):

- Are your shoulders rounded?
- Is your pelvis tilting forward?
- Are you slouching at your desk or when feeding?

Focus on the core four

Focusing on these muscle groups (the essential mum muscles) will protect your spine, reduce joint pain, and support long-term mobility.

1. **Transverse abdominis (deep core):** Engage your core by exhaling and drawing your belly gently inwards. Do this when lifting, bending, and walking.

2. **Glutes:** These are your powerhouse. Weak glutes = overloaded hips and lower back. Try bridges, clam shells, lunges, and climbing stairs.
3. **Rhomboids and postural muscles:** Undo the 'mum hunch' by strengthening your upper back with:
   • wall angels
   • rows with a resistance band or water bottles
   • reverse flies
4. **Pelvic floor:** Do your pelvic floor exercises daily (see page 90), but go slow – don't over-squeeze. Include both short and long holds.

Final Thoughts

Your body has done an incredible thing: it's adapted, compensated, and carried you through. Now, it deserves a little attention in return.

Whether you've just had a baby or you're 10 years into motherhood, your back and joints will thank you for a little extra care and attention. The truth is, you don't need a complex rehab plan or fancy equipment. You don't need perfect posture. You don't need a six-pack. You don't need to be anyone else's version of 'fit'. You just need to move with kindness, rebuild what's been weakened, and trust that it's never too late to feel better in your own body.

But, most importantly, be kind to yourself. Your body is healing. That tummy, that wobble, that stiffness – it's not failure. It's recovery in progress.

CHAPTER 6

'I'm Having Difficulty Concentrating'

LIFTING THE FOG AND REGAINING CLARITY

Have you ever walked into a room and forgotten why you're there? Or opened the fridge and stared blankly, unsure what you were looking for? Maybe you've lost your phone, only to discover it in your hand all along. If so, you're not alone.

I can't tell you how many times mums have sat in my consulting room, voices low, and said: 'Doctor, I feel like I'm losing my mind. I just can't concentrate anymore.' Some laugh it off as 'mum brain', others are terrified that it's something more sinister, like dementia. Almost always, there's shame – as if struggling to remember things means you're failing at motherhood.

Here's the truth: from the moment you become a mother, you carry a mental and emotional load unlike anything before. It's not just about feeding and caring for your child. It's about absorbing their needs, anticipating their emotions, managing the household, holding on to your work and identity, and somehow keeping yourself afloat in the middle of it all.

Motherhood reshapes your entire internal world. You go from thinking mainly about yourself to thinking about your child all the time – even when you're not physically with them. Your brain becomes constantly alert: *Are they OK? Do they need me? Did I sign that form? Why are they quiet?* That vigilance can be protective in that it helps keep your baby safe, but, over time, it becomes exhausting.

This isn't to scare you, it's to validate what you might already feel: that this mental fog isn't just 'in your head'. Maternal cognitive load is real. It's measurable. And it matters.

What the science says

We know from neuroscience that chronic sleep deprivation, fragmented attention, and persistent stress can affect key areas of the brain, such as the hippocampus and prefrontal cortex, which are responsible for memory, focus, and decision-making. In fact, long-term studies have shown that cognitive strain from chronic overload and poor sleep, particularly in women, may be linked to increased risks of depression, burnout, and even dementia later in life.[1] One study highlights that chronic sleep disturbance is associated with cognitive decline, memory loss, and increased risk of dementia, especially in women. Although it focuses on older adults, the mechanisms begin accumulating earlier in life and chronic sleep deprivation in motherhood is a key window where this cognitive strain builds.

Difficulty concentrating is one of the most common and most misunderstood parts of being a mother. From baby brain to perimenopausal brain fog, concentration struggles are part of the maternal journey. They're a sign that your brain and body are adapting to massive physical, hormonal, and emotional shifts while also carrying the invisible weight of family life – and sometimes that shows up as brain fog.

The Reality of Brain Fog

Do you feel like you've got 57 tabs open, your brain's running on 1 per cent, or that you're forgetful, fuzzy, and just not quite yourself? Perhaps you've read the same email three or four times, but your brain just won't register what it says. This is 'brain fog' and it's something that I see and treat a lot as a GP.

Brain fog is a relatively new term. When I was studying neurology at medical school, we learnt about the brain, but the lecture on 'mum brain' was definitely missing! Over the years, though, it's been used more and more, and I feel it encapsulates how many of my patients feel.

Brain fog is more common in women – I see it a lot in mums and those who've got carer responsibilities – but really it can affect anyone who is spinning all the plates at work and at home, and also dealing with general life and everything in between.

Brain fog is the product of that intense mental load that we've touched on throughout this book, and there are biological reasons behind why it happens, which can often be overlooked:

- **Low iron or vitamin B12:** This means that your brain cells don't get the oxygen or nutrients that they need.
- **Low vitamin D:** Vitamin D is essential for nerve signalling and your mood.
- **Underactive thyroid:** This can cause your brain to feel quite flat and sluggish.
- **Autoimmune conditions:** Conditions such as coeliac, lupus, or Hashimoto's can cause chronic low-level inflammation that can impact your brain health.
- **Poor sleep:** Sleep is when your brain clears out waste, files memories, and resets itself. Without enough quality sleep, your thinking becomes slower, attention span shorter, and memory patchier.
- **Chronic stress:** This causes spikes in your stress hormones that can affect your memory, focus, and mood.

- **Hormonal changes, especially during the perimenopause:** As oestrogen levels start to fluctuate and drop during perimenopause, many women notice brain changes well before any physical symptoms start.

It's worth bearing in mind, too, that alcohol and caffeine can both make brain fog worse.

Brain fog is more common in the months and years after having children and even more common during the peri/menopause, often triggering women to question whether they have premature dementia.

Brain fog creeps up on you and can feel like a big cloud that has come between you and your brain. It usually shows up as fuzziness around ordinary everyday tasks, memory changes, word-finding difficulties, easy overwhelm, processing difficulties, or simply just not feeling like yourself anymore ... At first it can feel funny – forgetting your kid's name or walking into a room and forgetting why you went in there – but as the pattern repeats itself, frustration seeps in.

If this is you, you are not 'just tired' – brain fog is a science-backed phenomenon and it is a signal from your body telling you that your battery is low and you need to charge up.

When to seek help

In most cases, mum brain is not dementia. It's due to fluctuating hormones, lack of sleep, stress, and mental overload – all of which can be treated or supported. If you're worried, here's how to tell the difference.

Mum brain is likely if:

- It began in pregnancy, postpartum, or perimenopause.
- It worsens when you're tired, stressed, or overloaded.
- It shows up in everyday life (forgetting keys, names, words), but not in safety-critical tasks, such as driving,

administering medicine, or managing work responsibilities that require precision.
- It fluctuates – you have some good days, and some foggy days.

See your doctor if:
- Symptoms are persistent and worsening.
- You get lost in familiar places.
- You struggle with tasks you've always managed (for example, cooking a familiar meal or paying the bills).
- It affects your ability to care for yourself or your children safely.
- There are other symptoms such as weight change, mood shifts, or neurological signs (like numbness, tingling, muscle weakness, changes in vision, or problems with coordination or speech).

Think about it: at every stage of motherhood, your brain is being asked to rewire itself – and it does, remarkably well. In pregnancy and postpartum, it prioritizes bonding and vigilance. In the school years, it adapts to hold huge volumes of logistical detail and prioritizes emotional labour and protection. And in peri/menopause, it shifts again, preparing for a new chapter of womanhood. Each transition has its challenges. Each comes with foggy moments. But each is survivable, treatable, and – with the right support – can even be transformative.

In this chapter, I'll take you through concentration and memory struggles across the decades of motherhood: the foggy early days, the overloaded school years, and the hormone-driven shifts of peri/menopause. Along the way, I'll share the science, my own story, and those of women I've cared for – and, most importantly, the things you can do to feel sharper, calmer, and more confident again.

Let's start with a phrase you've probably heard a hundred times: 'mum brain'.

'Is This Mum Brain?': The Baby Years

'Mum brain' (or 'baby brain') has become shorthand for forgetfulness: losing keys, mixing up words, or forgetting appointments. It's so entrenched that we joke about it. But the truth is, there's science behind it.

What the science says

As we saw in the last chapter, pregnancy and motherhood literally reshape the maternal brain.[2] This isn't brain damage. It's adaptation. These changes appear to fine-tune a mother's ability to respond to her baby's cues, strengthen emotional bonding, and sharpen vigilance. In other words, your brain is rewiring for motherhood. However, there is a trade-off. Your attention narrows towards your infant, which is brilliant for keeping them safe and attuned to their needs. The downside is that your memory and focus for other things – daily errands, names, where you put your phone – can slip more easily.
   Then add to that:

- **Hormonal shifts:** Oestrogen and progesterone plummet after birth, influencing serotonin, dopamine, and acetylcholine – neurotransmitters that are all key to mood and memory.
- **Sleep deprivation:** Even one night of broken sleep reduces attention as much as mild alcohol intoxication.[3] Now imagine months – and sometimes years – of it ...!
- **Nutrient depletion:** Iron deficiency, B12 deficiency, and thyroid dysfunction are all more common postpartum, and each can cause brain fog.

- **Emotional load:** This includes everything from processing birth trauma to the weight of being wholly responsible for another life.

No wonder so many new mothers find that their concentration scatters. A 2018 systematic review confirmed it: mothers report modest declines in memory and executive function during pregnancy and postpartum, though these usually improve with time.[4]

In my first year of motherhood, I once drove to the supermarket, did a full food shop, paid for it – and came home with an empty boot. My shopping was still sitting neatly bagged in in the trolley, in the car park, where I had stopped to talk to someone. Thankfully, it was still there when I got back. That wasn't carelessness. It was exhaustion. I was struggling with a baby with silent reflux, waking every 90 minutes in the night, trying to process a traumatic birth, and living with postnatal depression. My brain was saturated. Now, the funny thing was that my patient care always stayed sharp, because that part of my brain was switched on like a safety net. But in my 'mum life'? I forgot everyday things constantly. And that distinction matters because it shows that your brain isn't broken. You're not losing your intelligence or your capability. You're operating in survival mode, and your brain is prioritizing what it sees as most urgent. When you're constantly interrupted, overstimulated, and sleep-deprived, your working memory takes a hit, not because you're failing, but because your mental load is maxed out. That's a physiological response, not a personal flaw.

The role of sleep

As we explored in Chapter 2, sleep isn't just rest. It's maintenance. During deep sleep, the brain consolidates memories and clears out 'metabolic waste' through what is called the glymphatic system. This is a network of tiny channels in the brain that act like a night-time cleaning crew. During deep sleep, fluid washes through the brain, carrying away the waste products that build up while you are awake. If you get a good stretch of sleep, the bins are emptied and your brain feels clearer. However, if you are up every couple of hours with a baby, the bins don't get collected. The rubbish piles up and the result is that foggy, heavy, can't-think-straight feeling.

When sleep deprivation becomes chronic, especially over months or years, it's not just about feeling tired. It can begin to affect long-term brain function. We know that poor sleep impairs attention, decision-making, memory, and mood – all things that mothers rely on daily. It can even increase the risk of conditions like depression, anxiety, and cognitive decline later in life. The good news is, in most cases, this is a reversible state – not permanent damage. When sleep improves and your body is supported with the right nutrition, movement, and medical care, if needed, cognitive clarity usually returns. But that doesn't mean we should ignore it. Dismissing maternal brain fog as just 'what happens' after having kids does women a huge disservice – because it *is* a medical, and treatable, issue.

One mum who was four months postpartum came to see me, distraught. She'd left her laptop on the train – the third big lapse that month. 'What if I've got dementia?' she whispered. But she was breastfeeding round the clock, had returned to work, and was surviving on four hours of broken sleep. Her brain wasn't failing – it was exhausted. Once we worked on sleep support, her partner took over one night feed, and she gave herself permission to rest, the fog began to clear.

The nutrient factor

Many mothers are iron-deficient after birth, especially if blood loss was significant. Low iron reduces oxygen delivery to the brain, impairing concentration. Vitamin B12 deficiency can cause fatigue, poor memory, and even neurological symptoms. Thyroid changes (like postpartum thyroiditis) can also mimic brain fog. (See page 43 for more on the symptoms of vitamin and nutrient deficiencies.) These are treatable causes – but they're often missed because symptoms get written off as 'just being a mum'. I hear this so often and, honestly, it makes me furious. Why do we keep writing off women's symptoms as 'just part of motherhood'? Fatigue, brain fog, and poor concentration are not things you should have to simply endure. If a non-parent walked into a clinic with these symptoms, we'd investigate them properly. Mothers deserve that same level of care, attention, and respect.

What you can do

- **Delegate without guilt:** You are not meant to do everything alone. Sharing tasks isn't weakness – it's survival. If you have a partner, swap shifts so each of you gets some solo downtime. If you're parenting alone, lean on friends or family where possible, even for short breaks.
- **See your doctor:** Ask for bloods to check iron, B12, vitamin D, and thyroid if fog persists.
- **Prioritize micro-rests:** If long sleep isn't possible, even a 20- to 30-minute nap or quiet time in bed helps.

'There's Not Enough Time in the Day': The School and Teenage Years

If the newborn stage scatters your brain with hormones and sleep loss, the school and teen years scatter it with sheer logistics and emotional overwhelm.

The invisible work of motherhood – the remembering, the anticipating, the planning, the knowing when the dentist appointment is, that the red PE kit is for Tuesdays, that your child will only eat sandwiches cut diagonally, that the homework is due next Friday, and so on – really ramps up at this stage.

During the COVID pandemic, a report from the Institute for Fiscal Studies and UCL Institute of Education showed that mothers continued to shoulder twice as much unpaid childcare and housework as fathers – even when they both worked.[5] From what I see in clinic and hear anecdotally from friends, that imbalance hasn't gone away.

And, once again, there's science behind this mental juggle.

> ### What the science says
>
> Our brains can hold about four things in working memory at once.[6] Mothers are often juggling 14. Multitasking feels inevitable once you become a mum, but it comes at a cost: slower performance, more mistakes, and that constant sense of fog. That 'scatterbrain' feeling isn't weakness – it's neurological overload.

I've lost count of the number of times I've sprinted from surgery to the school gates, still half-immersed in patient care, with my mind also whirring through dinner plans, afterschool clubs, and a talk I need to prepare. On those days, it isn't that I can't concentrate, it's that there's no room to.

A mother of three similarly told me: 'By 9pm, I realize I've done everything for everyone else and nothing for me.' Her brain felt scattered and joyless. Once she decided to carve out two evenings a week just for herself – even just reading in bed – she felt sharper and calmer.

The teen years: A hidden cognitive load

By the time your children hit adolescence, you might expect that the concentration struggles of early motherhood would ease. But what many women discover is that their brains feel just as overloaded – sometimes even more so.

While the practical demands of motherhood change over time, the cognitive labour does not disappear – it simply takes on new forms, and mothers continue to carry the majority of the mental load involved in planning, anticipating, and managing family life, even as children grow older. Instead of nappies and nap schedules, it is worry about mental health, school performance, and safety. This invisible emotional vigilance drains focus just as much as broken sleep once did. You no longer have to remember which breast you last fed from, but you're now remembering exam timetables, social plans, Snapchat passwords, and who's fallen out with who this week. You might also be:

- monitoring for signs of anxiety, depression, or self-harm
- negotiating boundaries around social media, parties, alcohol, and dating
- providing emotional containment when they rage or cry
- lying awake at night, waiting for them to come home safely

Cognitive psychology tells us that working memory is limited. Add too many items, and performance drops. But this emotional labour – worrying, monitoring, anticipating – counts as cognitive load too.

It's a lot and I'm starting to feel it too. With my children older now, my brain sometimes feels hijacked by their feelings. When your child is struggling at school, or anxious about friendships, or arguing with you daily, your focus fragments. Even when I'm at work, a part of my brain stays tethered to them. That's motherhood – but it explains why our brains can feel foggy, even when we're technically 'past' the sleepless baby years.

If any of this resonates with you, take the nudge and book in with your doctor to discuss your brain fog. They will take a history and also do some blood tests to investigate the underlying cause and treat it accordingly.

> ## The cost of chronic overload
>
> Constant stress raises cortisol and chronically high cortisol affects the hippocampus, the brain's memory hub, impairing recall and learning. It also disrupts sleep, creating a vicious cycle. That's why overloaded mums often present with fatigue, IBS flare-ups, headaches, or skin rashes – their bodies are showing the strain.

What you can do

- **Protect your bandwidth:** Say no to draining commitments and ask your child open-ended questions ('What was the best part of today?') instead of interrogating them. It builds connection without overwhelming you.
- **Have a digital detox:** Screens aren't just draining for your eyes, they scatter your attention, eat into your downtime, and overload your brain with constant notifications, messages, and noise. Try creating small screen boundaries that work for your life: no phones at the dinner table, screen-free mornings, or even one evening a week off social media. You'll be surprised how much more present, calm, and connected you feel – both to yourself and your family.
- **Self-care is not optional:** Protect at least one piece of time each week just for you. Guilt-free.

'My Brain Feels Like Cotton Wool': The Peri/Menopause Years

Now let's talk about perhaps the most under-discussed stage of maternal brain health: peri/menopause. Here is what mothers describe to me in clinic:

- 'It's like I'm walking through fog.'
- 'I know the word, but it won't come out.'
- 'I read the same page three times and it doesn't go in.'
- 'I'm terrified it's dementia.'

These are phrases I hear almost daily from women in their 40s and 50s. The cruel thing is that many feel dismissed when they bring this up.

What the science says

Oestrogen is not just about reproduction – it's a cognitive hormone and it interacts with the neurotransmitters:

- acetylcholine (for memory and learning)
- serotonin (for mood and focus)
- dopamine (for motivation and reward)

During perimenopause, oestrogen levels fluctuate unpredictably, which disrupts these neurotransmitters. The result? Concentration, recall, and focus all feel impaired. One study showed measurable dips in processing speed and verbal memory during the menopausal transition,[7] and systematic reviews show that many women report subjective cognitive difficulties, such as memory problems and 'brain fog', during the menopausal transition, even when objective cognitive testing remains largely normal.[8]

For mothers, all this can feel particularly overwhelming. You're still holding the mental load – remembering school forms, birthday parties, dinner plans, and doctor appointments – all while navigating fluctuating hormones, disturbed sleep from night sweats, aching joints, and the emotional stress of parenting teenagers or caring for ageing parents. No wonder so many mums describe this phase as 'cotton wool brain' – it's not just forgetfulness, it's cognitive overload on top of chronic depletion. And yet, it's so often brushed off as 'just stress' or 'just ageing', when really, it's hormonal, neurological, and deeply real. Misdiagnosis leads to women being given antidepressants when what they may need is hormonal support. This dismissal also fuels fear. When I talk this through with patients and they realize it's perimenopause, I see the relief flood in.

HRT and brain fog

For many, HRT is life-changing. Let's take a quick look at what it can and can't do so you can decide whether it might be right for you.

What HRT can do:

- Stabilize oestrogen fluctuations, supporting neurotransmitters.
- Improve sleep by reducing hot flushes and night sweats.
- Indirectly boost concentration by improving mood and reducing anxiety.

What HRT can't do:

- Eliminate every concentration lapse.
- Guarantee sharper memory in all women – responses vary.

Talk to your family doctor about whether it's something you want to try.

The sandwich generation

Women aged 40 to 45 are the most likely to be caring for both children and ageing parents. Studies show this 'sandwich generation' reports the highest stress, lowest sleep, and greatest concentration difficulties of any group of mothers.[9] Functional MRI studies also show that every time we switch tasks, our brains use extra energy and take longer to return to baseline.[10] When you're caring in three directions at once, concentration fractures.

If this is you:

- Acknowledge it's not just you being disorganized – it's a real load.
- Speak to your family doctor if overwhelm is persistent.
- Access respite care and community services for elderly relatives where possible.
- Protect your own health appointments as fiercely as your family's. You matter too.

When it's something more

While brain fog during perimenopause is common – often linked to hormonal fluctuations, poor sleep, and the relentless mental load of motherhood – we must also acknowledge that other medical conditions can present with similar symptoms. And that's what can make this stage feel frightening.

Conditions such as underactive thyroid (hypothyroidism), vitamin B12 or iron deficiency, anaemia, chronic fatigue syndrome, fibromyalgia, autoimmune conditions like lupus or coeliac disease, and even long COVID can all cause symptoms like memory lapses, poor concentration, and mental fatigue. The overlap can make diagnosis tricky and leave many women fearing the worst. It's also why some mothers quietly worry about early-onset dementia and feel terrified to voice it.

While it's far less common than hormonal brain fog, early-onset Alzheimer's and other dementias (which typically present before age 65) do exist. They are rare but not unheard of, and the anxiety around this possibility deserves to be met with care, not dismissal.

So how do you tell the difference? Below are some signs that might suggest it's time to explore further medical investigation:

- You get lost in familiar places or struggle to follow familiar routines.
- You frequently forget the names of close family members or important details.
- You find it difficult to manage everyday tasks like cooking a meal or handling money.
- You notice significant changes in language, such as struggling with words or sentence construction.
- Others are noticing changes in your personality, judgement, or behaviour.
- Your cognitive symptoms are progressively worsening and don't vary day to day.

If any of this resonates, please don't panic – but do speak to your doctor. It's important that brain fog is taken seriously and investigated properly. Most of the time, we find a reversible or manageable cause (like hormone shifts or nutritional deficiencies), but if something more serious is going on, early detection can make a big difference.

One mum, a project manager, came to me devastated: 'I can't remember things I used to know. I've lost my sharpness. I think I'm getting dementia.' She was in perimenopause. Once we discussed her options, she started HRT, improved her sleep hygiene, and built regular exercise into her week. Within months, she reported that her focus and confidence had returned.

What you can do

- **Prioritize sleep hygiene:** Sleep can become challenging in the peri/menopausal years as low levels of hormones such as oestrogen, progesterone, and testosterone lead to low levels of the sleep hormone melatonin. So, sleep hygiene becomes even more important: try to prioritize a cool, dark room, stick to a consistent bedtime, and limit screens at least an hour before bed.

- **Embrace exercise:** Both aerobic exercise and strength training are important at this stage of life as they boost brain-derived neurotrophic factor (BDNF), which supports memory.
- **Consider medical support:** HRT can be transformative. NICE guidelines support offering it for symptom relief, including cognitive symptoms.[11] CBT or short-term medication – such as selective serotonin reuptake inhibitors (SSRIs), which can help with low mood, anxiety, and brain fog – may also be useful, especially if HRT isn't suitable. Or they can be used in conjunction.

'Mum brain' in a nutshell

- **It's scientifically proven:** Pregnancy, motherhood, and perimenopause all reshape the brain.
- **It's common:** Up to 60 per cent of women report concentration problems at some stage.
- **It's likely not dementia:** Most fog is due to changing hormones, lack of sleep, stress, or overload.
- **It's treatable:** Sleep support, nutrition, exercise, therapy, HRT, and self-care all help.
- **It's survivable:** With support, most women regain clarity – often stronger than before.

Punam's Prescription

Open up

Too many women stay silent, ashamed to admit their brain fog. The stigma means symptoms are dismissed as 'just stress' or 'normal mum life'. Telling your family doctor, your partner, or even a friend is powerful. It moves the fog from a private fear into something that can be supported.

Peer support groups – online or local – can also reduce isolation and the shame often associated with the menopause years. Remember: you are in this with every other mother who has ever lived. (See Chapter 9 for more on the importance of connection.)

Breathe through it

When your nervous system is overloaded, your breathing gets shallow and fast, and your brain struggles to concentrate. Simple breathing exercises signal your nervous system to switch out of 'fight-or-flight' mode, lower cortisol, calm the amygdala, and restore focus.

Try box breathing: inhale for four, hold for four, exhale for four, hold for four, and repeat for two minutes. This shifts your body into a state where clarity returns.

Eat for your brain

What you eat really does impact how clearly you think and how well you focus. Your brain needs steady fuel – not sugar spikes and caffeine crashes – to stay sharp. Prioritize protein in every meal to support neurotransmitter function (the brain's messaging system). Include omega-3-rich foods like oily fish, walnuts, flaxseeds, eggs, and full-fat yoghurt – these healthy fats are vital for brain cell structure and mood regulation. And don't forget your iron: leafy greens, lentils, lean meats, and fortified cereals help carry oxygen to your brain, preventing that sluggish, foggy feeling.

A varied, colourful diet not only boosts concentration, but can also help with memory and mental energy – which every mum needs more of.

Keep your brain active

Brains love novelty. Every time you learn something new, you lay down fresh pathways. This doesn't just mean doing a Sudoku every day (unless you enjoy that, of course) – it means anything that stretches you. Learn a language. Try pottery. Read outside your comfort zone.

For me, it was saying yes to *Strictly Come Dancing*. I had two left feet, no confidence on the dance floor, and every excuse to say no. But saying yes gave my brain a new challenge. I had to memorize choreography, coordinate my body, and push through fear. It was terrifying – and exhilarating. That experience reminded me, and I remind my patients of this too: we are not just mums. We are women who can surprise ourselves. And the brain thrives when we do.

Final Thoughts

When your brain is foggy, the temptation is to criticize yourself. But self-criticism makes focus worse. Self-compassion reduces cortisol, improves resilience, and clears space for concentration.

Know that your brain is not broken. It's adaptable. Thanks to neuroplasticity, you can strengthen focus and clarity at any age.

CHAPTER 7

'I'm Feeling Scared'

MANAGING FEAR, THE BABY BLUES, AND COGNITIVE CHANGES IN LATER LIFE

Motherhood is not a straight path. It's a winding, messy, beautiful, exhausting journey through different terrain. Some stages feel like a gentle stroll; others feel like climbing a steep hill in the rain with no map. But every stage, every decade, is survivable – and not just survivable, but rich with opportunities to know yourself more deeply, to connect more fully, and to live more intentionally.

And yet, for all the love and joy, there can also be fear. Fear that you're not doing it 'right'. Fear that you're not enough. Fear that you're losing the version of yourself you used to recognize. Gosh, fear – it's one emotion you're not prepared for before you embark on this colourful journey.

I've been a GP long enough to know that every mother carries her own unspoken worries. Some are fleeting, while others linger for years. I've also been a mother long enough to have felt most of them myself – in the tear-filled early weeks after birth, in the exhaustion of toddlerhood, in the identity shifts of the school years, and now in the hormonal unpredictability of perimenopause. This chapter is therefore for every mother who has ever thought: *I'm scared I can't do this. I'm scared I'm not coping. I'm scared of what's changing in me.* It's about those moments when you feel unsure or completely lost. I want to give you the science behind what's happening in your brain and body, the stories that prove you're not alone, and the practical tools that can help you find your footing.

And here's what I've learnt from my own experience and from sitting across from hundreds of other mums in clinic: feeling scared doesn't mean you're weak. It doesn't mean you're failing. It means you're human. You're in the middle of one of the biggest physical and emotional transitions of your life, and your brain is trying to find its new footing.

So, let's walk through that fear together – from the wobbly early weeks of new motherhood right through the decades.

'Why Am I Crying All the Time?'

Let's start at the beginning – those early days and weeks of motherhood when you're home with a newborn and everything feels … well, intense. I know how challenging these early days can be. Nobody prepares you for how much life will change and, as beautiful as this chapter can be, it can feel overwhelming.

First off, I want you to know that crying in those early days is normal, especially in the trying stages, the exhausting stages, the 'I don't know what I'm doing' stages – no matter who you are, it's OK! You've just done this monumental thing: grown and birthed a human. Whether it was a straightforward delivery or a rollercoaster of interventions, your body is now in recovery mode. Your hormones are recalibrating, you're operating on broken sleep, and you've got this tiny person who needs you 24/7. It's no wonder so many new mums cry. Most new mothers experience a mild, short-lived period of tearfulness, mood swings, and overwhelm in the first week or two after birth – often referred to as the 'baby blues' – and clinical estimates suggest this affects a majority of women, with many studies reporting rates up to around 85 per cent.[1] These are mild, short-term emotional changes – including tearfulness, mood swings, and anxiety – that usually settle within 10–14 days without any treatment. It's a normal adjustment phase as hormones shift and the realities of early motherhood set in.

The baby blues

If you've just had a baby and find yourself crying at TV adverts, weeping in the shower, or feeling on the verge of tears for no obvious reason, you are not alone and, no, this isn't a sign of weakness or that you're 'not coping' – it's biology. The baby blues are a physiological response to an enormous hormonal shift. Here's what's going on:

- **Hormones drop:** Oestrogen and progesterone – two key pregnancy hormones – plummet in the days after birth. These aren't gentle shifts; your levels can fall from some of the highest they'll ever be to some of the lowest, in just a few days. Oestrogen affects serotonin (your 'feel-good' brain chemical), and progesterone supports GABA (which helps keep you calm). When those hormones drop so suddenly, it's no wonder your emotional balance takes a hit.
- **Oxytocin surges:** This 'bonding hormone' spikes during and after labour, flooding your system to help with attachment and breastfeeding. But like any big hormonal wave, it can also leave you feeling weepy, overwhelmed, or wide open – especially in those first days and weeks.
- **Sleep deprivation:** Even a few nights of broken sleep can impact your brain's ability to regulate mood, manage emotions, and think clearly. It's a massive hit to your emotional bandwidth.
- **Overwhelm:** There's no manual for your baby. Every cry, feed, nappy, and wake-up is brand new. The mental load starts early – and the uncertainty can make it all feel even heavier.

And the result? You cry because the baby's awake. You cry because the baby's asleep. You cry because someone ate the last biscuit. This is all normal in those first couple of weeks.

The baby blues usually settle within two weeks, but if low mood, anxiety, or hopelessness continue, it might be postnatal depression (PND) or anxiety. These are common, treatable conditions, but too many women try to soldier through in silence.

When it's more than baby blues

I had PND after my first birth, but I didn't recognize it at first. I was a GP, so I thought I should be coping. Surely I knew what to expect? Surely I could logic my way through it? But mental health doesn't work like that.

After my first traumatic birth, my tears weren't just hormonal. They were tangled up with fear – fear that my body had failed, fear that I wasn't going to bond with my baby, fear that the deep exhaustion I felt would never lift. I remember sitting in my bedroom, blinds drawn, baby finally asleep, feeling utterly disconnected from the rest of the world. I knew, as a doctor, what the baby blues were supposed to look like. But this felt different.

It's estimated that nearly one in six mothers experience significant anxiety or depression in the perinatal period.[2] Postnatal depletion, chronic stress, perimenopause-related mood changes, and the sheer mental load of raising a family can play a huge part.

What makes it worse is that women often internalize it, assume it's 'just them', and wait until they're in crisis to get help. But feeling like this is not a reflection of your ability as a parent. PND and postnatal anxiety are medical conditions that deserve treatment and support, just like any other health issue.

PND can feel like:

- being persistently sad, flat, or tearful
- feeling guilty or like you're a 'bad mum'
- struggling to bond with your baby

- avoiding friends, family, or activities you used to enjoy
- feeling hopeless about the future

Postnatal anxiety can feel like:

- constant worry, often about the baby's safety
- racing thoughts you can't switch off
- physical symptoms like a racing heart, sweaty palms, or breathlessness
- panic attacks
- intrusive thoughts, distressing mental images, or urges you don't want

Research suggests that 70–100 per cent of new mothers experience intrusive thoughts about harm coming to their baby, such as imagining them slipping out of their arms, falling from a height, or not breathing in the night.[3] These thoughts can be deeply distressing, but are extremely common, especially in the early postpartum weeks, and are generally a sign of heightened anxiety and hypervigilance, not illness. You're not weird, broken, or a bad mum – you're human, and your brain is trying to process a huge life change.

With my first baby, I didn't sleep – even when he did. I'd lie awake imagining every possible disaster: choking, sudden infant death syndrome (SIDS), falling down the stairs while carrying him. I told myself I was being vigilant, but, really, I was on high alert 24/7, and it was exhausting. Looking back, I can see I was deep in postnatal anxiety as well as PND secondary to birth trauma. Yes, the two can co-exist, and I wish I had that insight sooner back then; hindsight is a great thing!

One mum I saw in clinic came in at six weeks postpartum. She told me she felt 'flat' all the time. She wasn't crying constantly, but she also wasn't laughing. She was going through the motions of feeding, changing, and rocking her baby, but she felt disconnected, like she was watching her life on TV. She thought maybe she was 'just tired' and needed to 'pull herself together'. In reality, she was experiencing classic PND. With the right support – talking therapy, practical help at home, and, for her, a short course of medication – her symptoms improved dramatically within a few months. I occasionally see her with her now seven-year-old with the odd sore throat, but, other than that, you would never know what they had been through back then.

What the science says

During the early postpartum period, your brain is undergoing structural and functional changes. MRI scans show that areas involved in empathy, emotion regulation, and motivation actually rewire themselves after childbirth.[4] This neuroplasticity helps you respond to your baby's needs, but it also makes you more emotionally sensitive – which is a strength when it's balanced, but can tip into anxiety or depression when combined with stress, trauma, hormonal volatility, or lack of sleep or support.

The good news is that this is manageable and treatable. That's why it's so important to raise awareness, so signs and symptoms can be recognized early, and support and treatment can be put in place to help you heal. If any of this sounds familiar to you, please don't suffer in silence. Speak to your doctor or your health visitor. You can also self-refer directly for talking therapy in many areas of the UK, or access support through organizations like PANDAS Foundation UK (Pre and Postnatal Depression Advice and Support) or the Maternal Mental Health Alliance. If your symptoms are more severe, or you find they don't improve, medication can be a safe and effective option – and it doesn't mean you've failed

For some women, it's an important bridge to help them feel like themselves again.

There *is* light at the end of the tunnel. You won't always feel this way. With the right care, support, and time, you will come through it and rediscover your strength again.

When to seek help

The baby blues usually appear between day three and day five after birth, peak quickly, and resolve within two weeks. You might feel tearful, irritable, or anxious, but you can still experience moments of joy and connection.

If your low mood lasts more than two weeks, feels overwhelming, or is getting worse, it might be PND or postnatal anxiety. If *any* of these symptoms appear, please speak to your doctor immediately or seek emergency support:

- feeling hopeless
- not enjoying anything
- having thoughts of running away
- feeling like your family would be better without you
- having thoughts of harming yourself or your child

If you recognize yourself here, please know you deserve help, and you will not always feel this way.

When the tears return

Research shows that women are at a significantly higher risk of experiencing depression or depressive symptoms during the perimenopausal transition than when they were premenopausal. Some cohort studies report that the likelihood of depressive episodes is around 1.5 to 2.5 times greater during this phase compared with earlier reproductive years, and large meta-analyses show that perimenopausal women have about a 40 per cent higher risk of depressive symptoms than premenopausal women.[5]

There are biological reasons for this. Oestrogen begins to fluctuate and eventually decline during perimenopause. This hormonal rollercoaster can destabilize your emotional state, lower your resilience, and affect sleep, energy, and even how you process stress. But it's not *just* about biology. As we've explored in previous chapters, this phase of life often collides with peak responsibility. You might be juggling teenagers or young adults at home, caring for ageing parents, managing a demanding career, or navigating relationship shifts. Many mothers in their 40s and 50s describe feeling emotionally saturated, pulled in all directions, and invisible in a society that rarely stops to check in on them.

If you're in this phase and finding yourself tearful, irritable, anxious, or flat, know this: it isn't weakness. It's a season of recalibration. You're moving through a major transition – hormonally, emotionally, and often spiritually too. The most important thing is not to dismiss your symptoms or write them off as 'just hormones'. Help is available – from HRT and talking therapies to lifestyle shifts that support your nervous system and emotional well-being. You *deserve* to feel like yourself again. This phase can be challenging, yes, but it's also a powerful gateway to deep transformation and self-understanding. You're not fading. You're evolving.

What you can do

- **Know your normal:** Jot down a few words about your mood each day; tracking your feelings can help you spot patterns and identify when you might need extra help. If you are immediately postnatal and the baby blues don't lift after two weeks, or if you're further down the line and you feel persistently anxious, hopeless, or detached, reach out to your doctor or health visitor.

- **Eat to steady your energy:** Protein and slow-release carbs, such as grains, legumes, and starchy vegetables like sweet potato, can have a positive impact on mood.
- **Get outside once a day if you can:** Daylight helps regulate your body clock, which will help your mood and, eventually, your sleep. I'm not talking about a 5k walk – a lap round the block with the pram counts, or even just two minutes standing by the door or walking on the grass with a cup of tea.
- **Rest when you can:** Even a few minutes lying down makes a big difference, helping to reduce cortisol (your stress hormone), improve circulation, support healing, and give your nervous system a chance to reset. In a phase of life where sleep is broken and stress is high, small moments of intentional rest can have a powerful cumulative effect on your physical and emotional well-being.

'I Haven't Got a Clue What I'm Doing'

No matter what stage we're at, us mums often feel like we're winging it – whether that looks like googling our baby's symptoms at 2am, comparing ourselves to other mums in the playground, or wondering how to deal with the many mood swings of adolescence. Motherhood doesn't come with a manual and it's time we normalized the uncertainties that crop up and reveal the many steps we can take to rediscover our confidence.

The baby years: Information overload

When I became a mum for the first time, I thought I'd done my homework: I'd read the books; I'd trawled through forums; I'd even watched YouTube videos on swaddling like some kind of antenatal ninja. And then my baby arrived.

He didn't follow the 'three-hourly feed' rule. He didn't nap for the prescribed 90 minutes. He didn't respond to the white noise machine I'd bought after reading a five-star review at 2am. And because every book seemed to insist there was a 'normal' pattern, I assumed the problem was me and him. Instead of questioning the rules, I tried harder to make us fit them. I still get upset when I think of that time because the result of that was crippling exhaustion, frustration, and the slow erosion of my confidence as a mother.

I'll never forget and always feel thankful to my mum for the day she recognized how much I was comparing and struggling. She said, 'Put the book down and read your baby.' Those words were so simple but so effective. She said my son may not have come with a physical manual, but he was constantly communicating to me if I listened to him, read his expressions, watched his cues, and felt him with my gut and heart. The books written weren't about him, or me, or us and our experience. We had our own journey and had to create our own routines that worked for us. This was hands down the best advice I have ever received – it changed my world in a single moment and I have shared it with countless mums since.

Now, I don't recommend burning books in the garden, but that's what I did that day. I had been at my wits' end and it felt like the most normal thing to do at the time. Burning those mummy books was freeing – a symbolic release from the idea that other people knew my baby better than I did. I was back in control. It changed everything from that moment, for the better.

Of course, it's completely natural to wonder if your baby is developing 'on time'. But comparison – especially in baby groups, chats with other parents, or online forums – can quickly spiral into quiet anxiety. You start hearing whose baby is sitting, crawling, walking, sleeping through … and suddenly it feels like a race. But babies aren't machines with identical timelines; they're individuals.

Most variations in milestone timing are entirely normal. Unless a healthcare professional has flagged a concern, it's OK – and healthy – to let your baby find their own rhythm. When we try to mould them into someone else's schedule, we risk increasing stress for everyone.

What the science says

Maternal sensitivity – your ability to notice and respond appropriately to your baby – is one of the strongest predictors of secure attachment and healthy emotional development. You cannot get this from a chart in a book. Excessive and conflicting information only increases maternal anxiety, and high anxiety interferes with your ability to read and respond to your baby's cues.[6]

Babies thrive best when their caregivers are responsive, not when they stick rigidly to a timetable.

The advice I always give to mums at this stage is, firstly, please stop comparing your baby to the ones in books or on Instagram. I mean it. Those 'average' routines? They're averages – and babies aren't averages; they're individuals. Secondly, like my mum told me, watch your baby, not the clock; read your baby, not the book! And finally, protect bonding time with your baby – think skin-to-skin, talking, rocking, or just holding them close. Bonding time isn't just for cuddles (though those are wonderful too) – it helps *you* get to know *your* baby. These quiet, connected moments build familiarity and trust, which, in turn, make it easier to recognize your baby's cues: when they're tired, hungry, overstimulated, or just needing a cuddle. The more time you spend in close contact, the more attuned you become – and that responsiveness is what helps babies feel safe, soothed, and secure.

The toddler years: The comparison trap

Social media can be brutal at any stage of motherhood, but, somehow, it feels more intense when you have a toddler. You see videos of toddlers making elaborate crafts or eating kale chips, while yours is drawing on the wall with a crayon and surviving mostly on beige food. Comparison can chip away at your confidence, but it's worth remembering that what you see online is the highlight reel, not the reality.

Comparison doesn't just steal joy, it seeds self-doubt. You start to question your instincts. You wonder if you're doing it 'right'. And, before long, you feel like everyone else has figured it out except you. That creeping feeling? That's imposter syndrome – and it's very common in motherhood. It can make even the most loving, capable mums feel like they're failing, especially when they're already exhausted, overwhelmed, and operating on little sleep and endless to-do lists. I've been there and so, if you are feeling all of this, you are not alone.

But here's the truth: no two families will ever have the same experience because no two children, circumstances, or mums are the same. What works for someone else may not be right for you, and that's OK. You are not failing just because your toddler doesn't nap at the 'right' time or because dinner was fish fingers again. Trust your instincts, trust your bond with your child, and remember – you are the expert on your child. Nobody online can replace that.

The school years: The emotional labour

The school years are often described as the 'easy' phase of parenting – your child can feed themselves, toilet themselves, and you can (in theory) sleep through the night again. But talk to any parent in the thick of it, and you'll hear a different story. While you're no longer up at 3am for feeds, you might be lying awake at night wondering how you're going to juggle work deadlines with sports day or replaying a conversation your child had about being left out at playtime.

This stage also introduces something new: managing your child's social and emotional world. You're no longer just keeping them alive – you're helping them navigate friendships, handle disappointment, and cope with challenges. It's emotionally draining. A bad day at school can feel almost as bad for you as it does for them. And if your child has additional needs, you might find yourself in meetings with teachers, chasing assessments, or advocating for extra support – all on top of your own work and home life. You're in constant 'response mode' – answering emails, helping with homework, arranging childcare – so it's no wonder you feel out of your depth.

When my children reached school age, I expected life to ease up. Instead, I found myself drowning in admin. One week it was World Book Day, the next it was a bake sale, then a sports tournament. My diary looked like a logistical military operation. I learnt the hard way that unless I carved out time for myself, it would simply never appear.

While there can be major life circumstances exacerbating the stress and load of motherhood, often simple interventions and strategies can help ease it just a touch to help you feel like you're not drowning in it all. If you have a partner, let them take full responsibility for a task without micromanaging – and, by this, I mean handing it over completely, from start to finish. That includes the planning, the decision-making, and the follow-through. For example, if your partner is in charge of dinner one night, that means they decide what to cook, shop for the ingredients, and actually make the meal – without you writing a shopping list, offering reminders, or stepping in with suggestions unless they ask. This can feel uncomfortable at first, especially if you're used to managing all the moving parts. But mental load isn't just about the doing – it's the constant thinking ahead, anticipating, and remembering that drains you. Sharing that load means letting someone else carry the whole thing, even if they do it differently from you. It might not look how you'd do it, but that's OK. Done is better than perfect. Start with one recurring task and practise stepping back. It's not about being hands-off forever, but about creating space in your mind so that everything doesn't fall to you. That's not laziness – it's load-shedding. It's teamwork.

One mum I saw in surgery came in with headaches, fatigue, and irritability. Her blood tests were normal. When we talked, it became clear that she was doing the mental management for her entire household – remembering birthdays, paying bills, scheduling car services, and tracking all the kids' activities. We discussed ways to delegate and use shared calendars so the mental load was more evenly distributed. Within a few months, her symptoms had improved.

Of course, this kind of delegation depends on having someone to delegate to. If you're parenting solo, don't have family nearby, or your partner isn't able or willing to contribute equally, this advice can feel frustrating or out of reach. You're not imagining it – the load is heavier when it's carried alone. In these situations, the most powerful thing you can do is reduce the overall load where possible: simplify meals, say no to extra commitments, or let go of perfection in non-essential areas. If there's space for it, consider calling in paid support or accepting help from friends or your wider community – remember, the mental load isn't something we were ever meant to carry alone.

Midlife motherhood: The teen years and beyond

By the time your children are teenagers, you may think the hardest part is behind you. No more night feeds or toddler tantrums. But, while you might assume that you've got the hang of this parenting thing by now, many women find that familiar feeling of 'I don't know what I'm doing' creeping back in.

Parenting stress doesn't just vanish once your children grow up – it evolves. Teenagers are navigating a messy, beautiful, and often turbulent time in their lives and, as their parent, you're right there with them. One day they need you intensely, the next they barely speak to you. That unpredictability can feel unsettling, especially if you're used to being their emotional anchor. And when you're supporting older children through school pressures, friendship worries, or big feelings – often while also managing younger siblings, work demands, and your own midlife changes – it's no wonder that your brain and body feel exhausted.[7]

If you're feeling pulled in all directions, or even like you're getting it wrong, take heart: this is one of the most demanding stages of motherhood, and you're not failing; it's all about adapting – again. Your role is shifting, not shrinking.

What you can do

- **Limit your 'information diet':** Choose one or two trusted sources, and accept that normal looks different for every child and family.

- **Celebrate your wins, mama:** None of us really know what we are doing with this parenting malarkey and most of us are just winging it – and that's normal. How are you meant to know what to do when you've never done it before? However, showing up every day and getting through the greatest challenge of raising a good human is something to be proud of! Even in the chaos, there are always moments that are joyous that can be celebrated. The laughter, the love, and the connection we get from our children – those moments really are precious, and practising gratitude for them helps to top up the cup.

- **If you're parenting teens, give yourself extra grace:** Teenagers are unpredictable – loving and open one day, withdrawn or prickly the next. This shift can feel like a rejection, but it's not – it's a normal part of their growing independence. If you're also juggling younger children or going through perimenopause yourself, the emotional and hormonal load can feel overwhelming. Be kind to yourself. Know that if you're feeling frayed, it's not because you're doing anything wrong – it's because you're doing so much.

- **Take one moment at a time:** Whether you're in the trenches of toddler tantrums or teen meltdowns, sometimes the kindest thing you can do for yourself is to take the day in tiny chunks. Acknowledge that parenting has seasons – some hard, some soft – and none of them last forever.

'Will I Always Feel Like This?'

If you've reached the point where you're asking yourself this question, I want you to pause for a moment and breathe. The fact you're even wondering this tells me something important: that you have been carrying too much, for too long, without enough support. This is not a reflection of your ability, it's a reflection of your load.

So many mums sit in my GP room, eyes full, voice trembling, saying some version of the same thing: 'I don't recognize myself', 'I'm not coping like I used to', 'Is this just who I am now?' I always say the same thing back, 'No. This is not permanent. But it is a sign you need support.'

The reality is that nothing about motherhood is fixed. Your stress levels change. Your hormones change. Your circumstances change. Your children change. You change. What feels overwhelming today won't always feel this way, but those feelings won't magically lift unless you have the right help, space, and care. The brain and body are designed to recover, but not in isolation.

Your brain has something called neuroplasticity, which means it can adapt and heal. Your nervous system can down-regulate. Your gut can recalibrate. Your hormones can stabilize, but none of this happens well if you're still in survival mode. You can't heal in the same conditions that made you unwell and you shouldn't have to. Instead, recovery and healing come from:

- rest (even tiny pockets of it)
- support (practical and emotional)
- connection (sharing the load, being seen)
- medical care when needed
- reducing the constant 'alert' state your body is in

Self-blame keeps many women stuck. So many mums I see believe they 'should' be coping better: 'I have a good family – why am I not happy?', 'Other people manage – why can't I?', 'I wanted this baby so much – does struggling make me ungrateful?' The truth is, motherhood magnifies everything – your love, your fear, your worries, your responsibilities. You are not meant to carry all of it alone. You are not designed to be the village. If you are feeling sad all the time, irritable, hollow, anxious, disconnected, or exhausted in a way that rest doesn't fix, do not ignore this. The sooner you speak up, the sooner things can get better.

Whether it's your family doctor, health visitor, partner, friend, or colleague, telling someone is the first step to breaking the cycle. Saying it out loud cuts through the isolation that makes everything feel heavier and opens the door to options like:

- lifestyle support
- talking therapy
- perinatal or menopause mental health teams
- medication
- HRT, if appropriate
- social support or community resources

You'd be amazed how quickly things can improve once you're no longer white-knuckling your way through it.

I promise you will not feel like this forever. This is not the final version of you. This is a tired, overwhelmed, stretched-thin version of you, and one who desperately needs a break, care, and compassion.

You deserve support. You deserve rest. You deserve to feel like yourself again. With the right help, you absolutely will.

What you can do

- **Don't wait until crisis point to seek support:** You don't need to be at rock bottom to deserve help. If you're struggling with low mood, anxiety, irritability, crying spells, sleep issues, or feeling disconnected, please make an appointment to see your family doctor. Try to do this as a face-to-face consultation. They can talk through options, rule out physical causes, and get you support early.
- **Nourish your body (and keep it simple):** Blood sugar crashes can mimic anxiety and worsen low mood so try to aim for:
  - regular meals
  - protein at each meal
  - a piece of fruit or nuts in your bag
  - a big glass of water every time you enter the kitchen
  Remember, this isn't about perfection. It's about fuel.
- **Reduce the mental load where you can:** The mental load is a major contributor to sadness and low mood. Small shifts can make a big difference. Try:
  - using shared digital calendars
  - having once-weekly family planning meetings
  - batch-cooking or repeating meals
  - letting your partner take full responsibility for a task (see page 173 for my tips on how to do this without micromanaging!)

If you're parenting without a partner, or with someone who isn't able to contribute equally – whether due to separation, shift work, or other circumstances – it's even more important to lighten the pressure where you can. That might mean creating simpler systems, accepting help from friends or community, or letting go of the idea that everything has to be done a certain way. This isn't about lowering your standards – it's about protecting your well-being so you can keep showing up, without burning out. You're doing more than enough. Remember, you don't have to carry all the invisible work.

Barriers to getting help

Many women struggle for far longer than they need to because asking for help feels frightening. In clinic, I see mums minimize, apologize, or wait until they're in crisis, not because they don't need support, but because the barriers to seeking help are real.

Here are some of the most common ones we need to name out loud:

- **Fear of being judged:** Worrying someone will think you're a 'bad mum' if you admit you're struggling. This fear keeps countless women silent.
- **Fear of losing your job:** Many mothers worry that if they disclose mental health struggles, their workplace will see them as less capable, less committed, or less reliable, especially in industries where women already feel pressure to 'prove themselves'.
- **Fear of having your children taken away:** This is one of the biggest unspoken fears. The truth is: seeking help *protects* your family. Honest conversations with a doctor, health visitor, or therapist do not trigger safeguarding concerns unless there is immediate danger, and asking for help is actually seen as a sign of strength and safety, not risk.
- **Feeling like everyone else is coping better:** Comparison silences you. When you believe you're the only one struggling, you're less likely to reach out even though the majority of mums experience these feelings at some point.

- **Not wanting to 'burden' anyone:** Many women put everyone else's needs above their own. The idea of adding one more thing to someone else's plate feels unbearable.
- **Mum guilt:** Guilt can sound like anything from, 'I'm not good enough' to 'This is the life I wanted, so why am I sad?' This guilt keeps women suffering alone.
- **Lack of time or childcare:** Even making a doctor's appointment can feel impossible when you've got children to juggle.
- **Cultural expectations:** In some cultures, motherhood is idealized and admitting difficulty feels like shame or dishonour. That pressure is enormous.
- **Not recognizing symptoms as *symptoms*:** Many women think their low mood, irritability, fear, detachment, or exhaustion is 'just motherhood', not realizing these are classic signs of overload or depression.

'I'm Scared of Change': The Peri/Menopausal Years

As we've seen throughout this book, the menopause doesn't just arrive with a fanfare and obvious symptoms – it can creep in quietly. And the years leading up to it – perimenopause – are when the real rollercoaster begins. One day, you're juggling work, kids, and life as usual; the next, you're wide awake at 3am, your patience is fraying, and you've forgotten the name of the colleague you see every morning. Every single day in my clinic I hear women describe this stage as if they've woken up in someone else's body.

This transition can last anywhere from four to twelve years. Hormone levels, especially oestrogen and progesterone, start to fluctuate wildly, and those shifts can affect almost every system in your body:

- **Brain:** Oestrogen plays a key role in mood regulation, memory, and sleep. Fluctuations can cause anxiety, low mood, brain fog (see page 153 for more on this), and insomnia.
- **Body:** You might notice joint aches (see Chapter 5), changes in weight distribution, new sensitivities to caffeine or alcohol, and temperature changes like hot flushes or night sweats.
- **Pelvic health:** Declining oestrogen can cause vaginal dryness, changes in discharge, recurrent UTIs, and reduced elasticity of pelvic tissues (see Chapter 3).
- **Cardiovascular health:** The protective effect of oestrogen on your heart starts to wane, making this a key decade for heart health awareness.

What the science says

Oestrogen has over 400 functions in the body and a huge number of them are in the brain. As we saw in Chapter 6 when we looked at peri/menopausal brain fog, it supports serotonin (for mood), dopamine (for motivation and pleasure), and acetylcholine (for memory and learning). When oestrogen fluctuates, those systems can go wobbly. Progesterone, meanwhile, has a calming effect via its interaction with the GABA system, which is like the brain's natural 'brake pedal', helping to quieten the mind and reduce overstimulation. Drops in progesterone – particularly in the second half of your cycle – can make you feel more anxious or restless. Testosterone also declines gradually, which can affect libido, muscle mass, and overall energy.

Why it feels so unsettling for mothers

Many women at this stage are still actively parenting teens or young adults, managing a household, and supporting ageing parents. Add fluctuating hormones, disrupted sleep, and mood changes, and it's no wonder so many mums feel like they're 'not themselves'. On top of all this, it can feel like the end of an era. Your reproductive years are coming to a close, and even if you weren't planning on having more children, it's completely normal to grieve that chapter. It's a big shift – physically, emotionally, and symbolically – and giving yourself space to process that is not only valid, but important.

For some, perimenopause feels like the emotional vulnerability of the early postnatal weeks – only now it's happening alongside bigger responsibilities and far less cultural acknowledgement.

The symptoms of perimenopause often get dismissed as stress, burnout, or even depression. So many women get disregarded, and that makes me both sad and just really mad – because I know it doesn't have to be this way. If you're feeling scared or worried about these changes, I want to reassure you that your body isn't broken. Your hormones are shifting and, as we've seen, that affects everything – your energy, your memory, your relationships, and your confidence. You're not just 'tired and stressed'. Perimenopause is science-backed, and it's powerful.

But I also know that change – especially when it's happening to your body and mind – can feel really frightening. You might not recognize yourself some days. You might feel like you're losing your spark, or questioning everything from your mood to your marriage. That uncertainty can be unnerving. Many women feel like they're coming undone, but what if you're not falling apart and instead you're evolving?

This is a transition into a new phase. A new identity. And while it takes time to figure out, you don't have to do it alone. You are still you – just shifting, growing, and becoming. And that's allowed to feel both scary and empowering all at once.

As I write this, I am right at the beginning of my own perimenopause journey. I've noticed the 3am wake-ups, the occasional word-finding pauses in conversation, the moments of unexpected irritability. Even with all my medical knowledge, I've had flashes of that same, 'What's wrong with me?' fear I felt after having my first baby. The difference now is that I know what's happening – and that makes it far less scary. And this is what I want for you too. My aim with this book is to give you the language, the knowledge, and the reassurance to understand what's happening in your body and mind, so that you never have to feel confused, alone, or blindsided by these changes. When we know the why, we can meet ourselves with more compassion. When we understand the science, we can stop blaming ourselves. And when we feel seen, we're far less likely to suffer in silence. You deserve to go through this next chapter of life feeling informed, supported, and empowered – not fearful or on the back foot.

The most important thing to remember is that there is help and support out there – whether that is lifestyle support, HRT, or just finally being heard. You deserve to feel like yourself again. We're in this together and, if you are struggling or fearing this change, I encourage you to make an appointment with your doctor (see my tips in the box overleaf to ensure you get the support and help you deserve and need).

What you can do

- **Do a self-audit:** Notice if low mood, anxiety, or exhaustion are constant. Don't ignore new symptoms – track them and see your doctor if they persist. The sooner perimenopause is on your radar, the sooner you can explore support options. That might include HRT, non-hormonal medications, or lifestyle changes tailored to symptom relief.
- **Bring your family on board:** Explain what's happening physically and emotionally so they understand that mood changes or fatigue aren't personal.
- **Reconnect with yourself:** This is a time of shifting roles and identities: children growing up, careers changing, and bodies transforming. Try carving out space to rediscover the parts of you that may have been quiet for a while – whether that's through journaling, joining a new class, revisiting an old hobby, or simply asking yourself, 'What

do I want now?' You're not who you were, but that's not a loss, it's a becoming.

- **Consider therapy:** Peri/menopause, especially alongside motherhood, is an emotional rollercoaster that can bring up all sorts of thoughts and feelings. If you are struggling, it's worth considering getting some therapy. Having someone who is impartial and trained to support psychological healing is an investment most people underestimate the value of.

How to talk to your doctor about peri/menopause

If you're feeling overwhelmed, low, foggy, anxious, sleep-deprived, or simply not like yourself, and you suspect it might be peri/menopause, please don't wait until things get worse. Make an appointment with your doctor. You don't need to have all the answers – just showing up and saying, 'I'm not coping' is enough. Here are some helpful tips to make sure you get the support you need.

Before your appointment, jot down:

- A rough timeline of your symptoms: when they started, how often they occur, and how they're affecting your day-to-day life (for example, work, sleep, relationships, memory, mood).
- Any changes in your periods or new physical symptoms like joint pain, hot flushes, or headaches.
- Mood-related changes like tearfulness, anxiety, irritability, panic attacks, or loss of motivation.
- Any concerns you have around brain fog, memory, or concentration (these are common).
- How your sleep has been and whether you're waking through the night.

- Any family history of mental health conditions, menopause-related issues, or hormone-sensitive illnesses.

What to ask your doctor:

- Could this be perimenopause or menopause?
- Should we check my hormone levels or bloods to rule out anything else?
- What lifestyle changes could support me?
- Am I a candidate for HRT and, if not, what are the alternatives?
- What are the benefits and risks of HRT in my case?
- Would CBT or another talking therapy help me?
- Are there any short-term medications that might help with sleep, anxiety, or low mood while I get back on track?
- Is there a local women's health or menopause clinic I can be referred to?

What support your doctor might offer:

- A clinical assessment and blood tests to rule out thyroid or iron deficiency (which can mimic perimenopausal symptoms).
- Advice on diet, movement, and sleep routines that support hormone and mental health.
- HRT options (patches, gels, tablets, combinations).
- Non-hormonal options (for example, SSRIs or serotonin–norepinephrine reuptake inhibitors (SNRIs) for mood or hot flushes if HRT isn't suitable).
- Referral for CBT, counselling, or talking therapy.
- Signposting to pelvic health physios, local women's groups, or menopause specialists.

Punam's Prescription

Speak about it

Silence is a heavy burden. Whether it's tears in the newborn stage, burnout in the school years, or mood changes in perimenopause, talking to someone and telling them that you feel scared lifts the weight. That could be your partner, a friend, a doctor, a counsellor, or even another mum at the school gate.

Stay connected

Isolation can amplify anxiety and low mood. Whether it's friends, family, or support groups, stay plugged into your community – it's more important than ever. Connect with other (like-minded) parents in the same boat. Whether it's a toddler group, a WhatsApp chat, or a friend who won't judge you for the mess in your kitchen, having someone to vent to makes all the difference. (See Chapter 9 for more on the importance of social connection.)

Eat to steady your energy

When everything else feels up and down – your mood, your sleep, your hormones – the simple act of eating regular, nourishing meals can help you feel more grounded. Protein and slow-release carbs, like grains, legumes, and starchy vegetables such as sweet potato, don't just keep blood sugar stable – they also support your brain chemistry, which helps steady your mood and anxiety levels. When your body feels nourished, your mind often follows. And in a time of change, that kind of steadiness can be deeply reassuring.

Check in with your sleep

You don't need perfect sleep, just better sleep. Try to:

- nap when truly exhausted (not instead of night sleep)
- avoid caffeine after 2pm
- prioritize an earlier bedtime
- introduce a wind-down routine before bed
- limit scrolling at night
- keep your bedroom cool and dark

Final Thoughts

If there's one thing I want you to take from this chapter, it's this: you are not failing. You are going through seasons – and seasons change.

From the weepy, sleepless haze of the newborn weeks to the chaos of toddlerhood, the calendar-clogging school years, the emotional shifts of midlife motherhood, and the hormonal rollercoaster of peri/menopause, each decade of motherhood brings its own unique challenges. It's not about 'getting back to normal' – it's about finding your new normal at every stage, and giving yourself the same compassion you give your children.

Remember: this is temporary. Your hormones, sleep, mental load, and life circumstances will shift. What feels scary today won't feel like that forever. I promise.

Fear is part of the wiring that keeps you showing up, day after day, for your children. It's also part of what makes you human. The real work – and the real freedom – comes from learning to live with that fear without letting it run the show. That means asking for help, resting without guilt, saying no to what drains you, saying yes to what sustains you, and knowing that every stage of motherhood comes with both its shadows and its light.

You are not alone. I'm right here with you – as a doctor, a mum, and a fellow traveller through all these seasons. And if no one has said it to you lately: you are doing better than you think.

CHAPTER 8

'I Feel Like I'm "Always On"'

REDUCING STRESS, SPOTTING BURNOUT, AND RESTORING YOUR RESERVES

From the moment we conceive, mums are 'always on'; forever tuned into the needs of our children, no matter how old they get. Even when we're lying in bed, our minds are flipping through the next morning's schedule, the forgotten birthday card, the washing that needs to be moved, or the worry our child shared at bedtime that we haven't stopped thinking about. My mum used to say to me, 'You'll understand when you have your own' – she was always there, always ready, always 'on' because she was so consumed in what my sister and I were doing. I understand it now … I am always 'on' too.

From a clinical perspective, we know this invisible load has a physical effect on the body. The constant stress activation – the mental load, the multitasking, the emotional labour – raises cortisol levels throughout the day. In short bursts, cortisol helps you cope. In long stretches, however, it grinds you down. When the 'on' stays on too long and the 'off' slips away, your nervous system begins to teeter …

Stress and its Impact on the Nervous System

Over time, chronic stress demands a lot from our autonomic nervous system (ANS), which controls the body's automatic functions, such as our heart rate, breathing, digestion, sweating, and blood pressure. The ANS is split into:

- **The sympathetic nervous system (SNS):** This is the 'on-your-toes' mode: quickening the heart, diverting blood to your muscles, releasing adrenaline and cortisol.
- **The parasympathetic nervous system (PNS):** This is the 'calm, digest, repair' mode: slowing the heart, stimulating digestion, allowing recovery.

The ANS is a finely balanced seesaw. When a threat appears, the SNS kicks in: your heart races, breathing becomes shallow, and muscle tone increases. That's the classic fight-or-flight response. Then, ideally, once the threat passes, the PNS presses the brake and the body returns to baseline. However, stress and motherhood tip that balance.

The hypothalamic–pituitary–adrenal (HPA) axis (which links the brain, adrenal glands, and stress hormones like cortisol) becomes hypersensitive when stress is sustained. Over time, if the PNS cannot catch up (for example, you're not getting quality rest, your digestion is suppressed, and your heart rate stays elevated), you become more vulnerable to anxiety, low mood, poor digestion, sleep problems, immune changes, and that 'wired but tired' fatigue we talked about in Chapter 2.

Nature designed mothers to be alert so their babies stay safe, but, in modern motherhood, where you often parent without the support of a larger community, that same hypervigilance can make you feel anxious, on edge, emotionally brittle, and utterly overwhelmed. It's not all in your head. Your nervous system has become the family radar – and it is always switched on.

When you're exhausted, when you're juggling a dozen demands, when you're touched out, when you're overstimulated, or when you're responsible for too much, your nervous system shifts into a state of 'fight or flight' far more easily. That's why you feel:

- irritated by normal noise
- unable to think clearly
- overwhelmed by small decisions
- tearful without knowing why
- anxious about asking for help
- guilty for not coping

Persistent SNS activation means that you are in survival mode more than you are in rest mode. Your nervous system hasn't had the chance to recover, and this affects mood regulation, memory, concentration, and physical health. Our bodies are built for short bursts of 'on' and longer periods of 'off'. Motherhood often flips that to long stretches of 'on' and short windows of 'off'.

What the science says

Studies show that the structural brain changes that happen during pregnancy, particularly in areas linked to empathy and social cognition, can persist for at least six years.[1] This means your brain stays primed for high sensitivity to all your child's needs, which is wonderful for connection, but can also mean you're more susceptible to stress when they're struggling.

It's easy to assume that once the baby years are behind you, your nervous system will go back to normal, but motherhood changes us in ways that last well beyond the early years. The good news, though, is that your nervous system can bounce back, but it needs you to stop, listen, and give it what it needs. You don't need to wait till you're 'broken'. You deserve recovery now.

In this chapter, I'll walk you through how stress builds, how to spot the early signs of burnout, and what you can do to protect yourself and rebuild your reserves. Because let's be honest: motherhood is beautiful but it is also relentless. From sleepless newborn nights to juggling school runs, work emails, and your teen's latest drama, the pressure never really lets up. You're always 'on' – mentally, emotionally, and physically. And while a bit of stress is normal (even helpful), when it becomes chronic, it starts to wear you down.

You might feel snappy, wired, weepy, or just plain exhausted – like you're running on fumes. And the worst part? You probably think it's just you. It's not. This is a pattern I see in my clinic all the time. Maternal burnout is real – but it's also reversible.

'I'm So Stressed All the Time'

This is something I hear from mothers in clinic on an almost daily basis. Too often, though, women's nervous system dysregulation goes unrecognized and is frequently dismissed as 'Just tired', 'Just stressed', or 'That's motherhood'. The result of dismissing women's feelings like this is:

- **Chronic stress:** This becomes toxic to the brain and body as elevated cortisol over time harms memory centres like the hippocampus, weakens immune function, disrupts sleep, and increases the risk of mood disorders.
- **Digestive issues, headaches, hormonal imbalances, and fatigue:** Symptoms like this often follow the unrelieved load.
- **Mothers reaching crisis point before intervention occurs:** When help is delayed, recovery is too.
- **A hidden cost to children and families:** A mother

under persistent nervous system strain cannot engage at the same emotional or physical level as one whose nervous system is supported. Once again, the health penalty rears its head and has an impact on both mothers and their families.

Often, in response to this nervous system overload, mothers adopt unhelpful coping strategies, such as:

- **Constant multitasking:** This keeps the SNS high and the PNS low.
- **Skipping meals, irregular sleep, and reliance on caffeine:** Unhelpful habits like this can stimulate the SNS further.
- **Neglecting your own needs:** Staying in go-go-go mode all day every day leads to chronic stress.
- **Ignoring emotional signals (because you 'should' be coping):** This means stress accumulates without being addressed.

In addition, you might find yourself:

- **Telling yourself 'You're just being dramatic' or dismissing your symptoms:** This only adds guilt and increases stress.
- **Waiting until 'everything else is sorted' to take care of yourself:** In fact, taking care of you positively affects everything else.
- **Thinking you must do it all alone:** Nervous system recovery depends on community, shared load, and rest.
- **Ignoring digestion, sleep, rest, and movement:** These are not optional in the nervous system recovery equation.

In the pages to come, we'll explore helpful strategies that will engage the PNS and reduce SNS activation at every stage of your motherhood journey.

The shock of the baby years

The baby years are beautiful, but they can also feel brutal. They're soft, warm, milky, and magical, but they're also some of the most stressful months of a woman's life. These are the years when your nervous system is in overdrive: there are new routines, disrupted sleep, unpredictable feeds, birth trauma, and hormonal fluctuations. All these raise baseline SNS activity and suppress PNS recovery. And yet most mothers are told, 'Enjoy every minute.' No wonder you end up stressed!

There are several reasons why the baby years are so stressful:

1. Sleep deprivation isn't just tiring; it changes your brain
In early motherhood, the frontal lobes, which are the parts of the brain responsible for planning, memory, and emotional regulation, function differently due to chronic lack of restorative sleep. Even moderate sleep loss affects:

- patience
- mood
- memory
- concentration
- appetite
- decision-making
- pain tolerance

And when you're waking every two to three hours (or every 45 minutes …!), you don't get the deep, slow-wave sleep your brain needs to reset. That's why new mums often feel:

- foggy
- tearful
- irritable
- forgetful
- more anxious

This isn't weakness. This is biology doing its best on too little fuel.

2. The hormonal rollercoaster is real

We've seen that, after birth, your levels of oestrogen and progesterone drop dramatically. Combine this with prolactin (drives milk production but can lower dopamine, affecting motivation), oxytocin (the connection hormone, but fluctuates with stress), and cortisol (often raised because of sleep disruption), and your emotional baseline becomes much more sensitive.

3. Feeding stress is huge!

Whether you breastfeed, bottle-feed, or combination-feed, feeding a newborn is intense.

Breastfeeding challenges alone – cracked nipples, mastitis, latch issues, tongue-tie, low supply, high supply – are a major reason for why so many new mothers feel stressed in the early weeks. And if feeding doesn't go to plan, which it often doesn't, the guilt can feel immense.

In my experience, bottle-feeding mums feel judged, breastfeeding mums feel pressured, and combination-feeding mums feel like they're failing at both. But the truth is: fed is best. Supported is essential.

4. The emotional load hits instantly

You suddenly become the keeper of:

- feeds
- sleeps

- nappy counts
- appointments
- development worries
- safety concerns
- household responsibilities

Your brain is doing the work of several separate jobs while operating on half a tank.

5. Comparison steals your peace

Social media, baby books, online forums, which are all full of 'shoulds' – 'Your baby should be sleeping X hours', 'Your baby should be self-settling', 'Your baby should be in a routine' – are exhausting. But we fail to remember that no two babies are the same. What you're reading is not your child. Meanwhile, your nervous system is constantly scanning, thinking, worrying – 'Am I doing this right?', 'Why is my baby crying?', 'Why am I not coping better?' Stress thrives in that environment.

I once saw a mum who came in already apologizing: 'I know you're busy, I'm probably overreacting but I'm just not coping.' She had a six-week-old with reflux, a toddler at home, a pelvic floor still recovering from birth, and a partner working nights. She thought she 'should be' handling it, but she wasn't sleeping, wasn't eating regularly, and felt she was shouting at her toddler constantly. Nothing was wrong with her, but, from listening to her, everything was wrong with her load. We talked about:

- splitting night shifts
- lowering expectations
- asking for family help
- safe co-sleeping
- planning one protected rest period during the day
- making feeding comfortable instead of ideal

Within a month, she came back for a review and said, 'I feel like myself again. I didn't need a different baby. I needed support.' This is true of so many mothers I see in clinic.

The chaos of the toddler years

The toddler stage is loud, messy, and full-on. You're chasing small humans with boundless energy while still dealing with sleep disruption, meal battles, and (often) returning to work. For mothers, this is a time when that 'always on' feeling can turn into burnout if self-care is constantly postponed. (We'll look at burnout in more detail on page 208.) Toddlers test boundaries to feel safe, which can make you feel like you're continually firefighting. It's also a stage when many mothers have their second (or third) baby too – layering pregnancy and postpartum recovery on top of toddler parenting.

From a brain perspective, your child is going through massive neural development at this time, especially in areas that control emotion and impulse, which is why meltdowns can be so intense. Toddlers are like little scientists in a permanent state of experimentation. The prefrontal cortex, which is the part of the brain responsible for self-control, decision-making, and regulating emotions, is still very immature at this stage. The limbic system, which controls emotional responses, is more developed, meaning emotions are big and intense, but self-regulation is almost non-existent. This is why a two-year-old can go from giggling to full meltdown in 30 seconds because their crayon broke in half. And because toddlers don't yet have the words or perspective to explain what's wrong, they use behaviour to communicate. For parents, that constant emotional intensity can feel like walking through a minefield.

For mothers especially, this is a stage when your patience is tested daily. You're often still recovering from the physical toll of pregnancy and birth, perhaps managing work commitments, and now you're negotiating with a small person whose logic changes hourly. Understanding that these behaviours are developmental, not personal, can help you stay calmer, but that doesn't mean it's easy when you're running on fumes.

Another reason this stage is so mentally demanding is the sheer load we've discussed in previous chapters. You're still managing your child's basic needs, but now you're also juggling nursery drop-offs, work schedules, and meal planning. The mental checklist never stops.

As a result of all these pressures, your stress hormones – particularly cortisol – can spike repeatedly during the day. Over time, without breaks or support, that chronic stress can wear down your resilience and leave you more vulnerable to anxiety, low mood, and burnout. It also leads to chronic inflammation within the body which, too, has long-term consequences.

What the science says

When left unchecked, chronic inflammation has been linked to a higher risk of a range of health conditions including heart disease, type 2 diabetes, autoimmune disorders, and even cognitive decline in later life. For mums, this means that the constant, low-level stress you carry now doesn't just affect your mood or energy, it can silently impact your long-term physical health, too.

Chronic inflammation is like a slow-burning fire in the body. When your stress response is constantly activated, whether from sleep deprivation, emotional load, or juggling everyone's needs but your own, your body keeps releasing stress hormones like cortisol. In short bursts, this is helpful. But over time, high cortisol levels lead to a cascade of physical effects: raised blood pressure, disrupted blood sugar regulation, and increased inflammatory markers in the bloodstream. Over years, this persistent inflammation can:

- **Increase your risk of cardiovascular disease:** Inflammation plays a role in the development of atherosclerosis (narrowing of the arteries), raising the risk of heart attacks and strokes.
- **Disrupt insulin sensitivity:** This increases the risk of type 2 diabetes.
- **Weaken the immune system:** This means that you recover more slowly and you are more susceptible to infections.
- **Exacerbate musculoskeletal pain:** This is particularly felt in the joints and muscles, which many mums already struggle with.
- **Affect cognitive health:** Long-term inflammation is linked to conditions like depression, anxiety, and, in later life, even dementia.

So, it's not 'just stress'. It's a physiological burden on your body. And it's why protecting your well-being now – through rest, nourishment, support, and boundaries – isn't a luxury. It's vital prevention.

One mum came to see me worried that she was 'shouting too much'. She had a three-year-old and a baby, no local family support, and a partner who worked long hours. She felt constantly guilty, convinced she was 'ruining' her children. She was simply stretched beyond capacity. We talked about the concept of a 'parenting pause' – stepping out of the room for 30 seconds to breathe before responding and how small breaks could help her reset. Within weeks, she noticed she felt calmer and more in control during those testing times. (See page 201 for 'What you can do' to relieve the stress.)

The mental load of the school years

When your child starts school, the demands shift. You become the keeper of the calendar, you know when the PE kit needs washing, when the school trip permission form is due, and when it's your turn to send in cupcakes (I've always just bought them!). For many mothers, this is also the decade when career responsibilities grow, ageing parents need more support, and social expectations pile up.

Chronic stress can lead to sleep problems, anxiety, and even physical symptoms like headaches or digestive issues. We saw in Chapter 6 that women still carry most household and childcare tasks, even when both parents work. This constant juggling can drain your mental bandwidth and make it harder to notice your own needs.

Then there's the ongoing sleep disruption. Even if you're not being woken up for night feeds, many parents in this stage still get less than the recommended seven to nine hours of sleep. Early mornings for school runs, evenings spent catching up on chores, work deadlines, and the mental churn of worrying about your child can all chip away at your rest, and chronic partial sleep deprivation can significantly impact mood regulation and your level of resilience.

I saw a 38-year-old mum who came to see me not because she was 'depressed', but because she was 'snapping all the time' and feeling like she had no patience left. She had two kids in primary school, worked full-time, and was constantly running late for something. She was eating lunch at her desk, skipping exercise, and staying up late to get a bit of quiet time after the kids were in bed. Gosh, I thought to myself – sounds so familiar! We talked about stress and how it can creep in slowly, especially when you're not making time for rest. She started by protecting one evening a week just for herself, even if it was just a bath and an early night. She also spoke to her boss about introducing more flexible working arrangements and joined forces with other parents for school pick-ups and drop-offs. It didn't fix everything, but it gave her some breathing space and, with that, came a bit more patience.

The shift in the teenage years

Motherhood in the teenage years can stir up a surprising amount of anxiety. You might find yourself lying awake at 1am wondering whether your teen is safe at a party, or worrying about exam stress, or second-guessing how much independence to give them. The emotional and logistical load is huge in this stage. It's no surprise that studies show higher rates of chronic stress, anxiety, and burnout in women in their 40s and 50s compared to men of the same age.[2] The toll isn't just mental; chronic stress raises blood pressure, disrupts sleep, weakens the immune system, and can even affect memory.

You might also be part of the 'sandwich generation' that we looked at on page 154, where you are caring for teens and ageing parents while also trying to keep your own career and health on track, which all keeps the SNS activated.

What you can do

- **Guard your downtime and plan joy:** The school calendar, work deadlines, birthday parties, and endless WhatsApp groups will swallow your time whole if you're not intentional. So, block out downtime before the diary fills up. Treat it like any other commitment because it is. Even one evening a week to rest, connect with a friend, or do something that brings you joy (yes, even if it's just a cuppa in silence or bingeing your favourite show) is protective for your mental health. Joy doesn't have to be big or expensive. It just has to be yours. A walk without your phone. Singing in the car. Ten minutes with a good book. Plan it. Prioritize it. Because if you wait for spare time to appear, it won't.

- **Keep moving:** Regular exercise isn't about 'bouncing back', it's about keeping your mood stable and your stress hormones in check. Even a brisk 20-minute walk after dropping off the children can help.
- **Watch for signs you need support:** Constant irritability, low patience, and feeling detached from your children are all signs you need a break – not because you're failing, but because you're human. Reach out to your family doctor for support.

'My Digestion Has Gone Haywire'

One thing I see again and again in clinic, and I'm sure many of you reading this will recognize, is how quickly stress shows up in the gut. You can be coping, coping, coping, and then, suddenly, your stomach is in bits: bloating, cramps, nausea, diarrhoea, constipation, acid reflux, or a miserable cycle of all the above. It's no coincidence.

What the science says

Your gut and your brain talk constantly through what's called the gut–brain axis. I often describe this as a two-way motorway: the brain sends signals to the gut, and the gut sends signals back. Your gut has its own nervous system – the enteric nervous system – which is why it's sometimes called the 'second brain'.

When you're stressed, especially when that stress is chronic, the body pumps out cortisol and adrenaline. These hormones divert blood away from the digestive system because, in fight-or-flight mode, digestion is not a priority. That's fine in short bursts, but when you're living in that stressed state for weeks, months, or years without proper recovery, the

digestive system becomes hypersensitive and sluggish.
That's when symptoms start to appear:

- bloating (your gut motility slows down)
- cramps (your gut muscles become overactive)
- loose stools (stress speeds things up)
- constipation (or slows them down)
- reflux and heartburn
- IBS flare-ups
- nausea
- appetite changes (either constant hunger or no appetite at all)

There is another layer too: gut microbiome changes. When you're stressed, sleeping poorly, eating irregularly, skipping meals, or relying on quick carbs and caffeine, the balance of bacteria in your gut can shift. Research shows that chronic stress can reduce diversity in the gut microbiome, and that can worsen both digestive and mental health symptoms.[3] It's a cycle: stress affects the gut, the gut affects the brain, and round and round it goes.

For mothers, gut symptoms often begin during periods of intense mental load – the baby years, toddler chaos, school schedules, the teenage emotional rollercoaster, and again in peri/menopause when your stress threshold narrows.

A mum once told me her anxiety was 'living in her stomach', and she was totally right. Many women feel their emotions in their gut before they feel them anywhere else. Butterflies, knots, heaviness, churning – they're all your body's early warning system saying, *Help, I'm overwhelmed.* You're not 'too sensitive'. Your gut is simply responding to your life and, in motherhood, that life is often a lot.

The good news is that gut symptoms caused by stress often improve dramatically when we support the nervous system (see my tips below).

What you can do

- **Eat regular meals:** Skipping meals or grazing all day can wreak havoc on your blood sugar, energy levels, and mood. You don't need to whip up anything elaborate – just aim for three nourishing meals a day with some protein, slow-release carbs, and plenty of fibre (think oats, wholegrains, pulses, veggies). This steadies your energy, supports your gut, and reduces those jittery highs and crashing lows that come with erratic eating.
- **Stay hydrated:** Your brain and body both function better when you're well-hydrated. Aim for around six to eight glasses of fluid a day (more if you're breastfeeding or very active). Water is great, but herbal teas, milk, and soups all count too. Dehydration can make you feel tired, sluggish, and more irritable – and it's one of the simplest things to fix.
- **Consider supplements or medical support:** For some women, probiotics, magnesium, peppermint oil, CBT for IBS, or medication if symptoms are severe are all valid options.

'I Can't Do It All'

If I had a pound for every time a mother has said 'I can't do it all', while exhausted, or defeated, I'd be able to fund maternity leave reforms myself. The phrase often comes out slowly, like a confession. What breaks my heart is that women always say it with shame, as though they've somehow failed at the job of motherhood when the reality is the opposite: you can't do it all because it is too much for any human being. The task is too big for one person; it was never meant to be a 'one-person job'.

When I hear a mum whisper this, I often think about what professor of psychiatry Dr Dan Siegel terms the 'window of tolerance' – the zone in which your nervous system feels safe, regulated, and able to cope.[4] Mothers in the so-called 'blue zone' are those who are well supported: they can process emotions, respond calmly to challenges, and rebound from stress. But most of the mums I meet? They're operating in the 'grey zone' – stuck between hyper-alertness and burnout. This happens when the demands placed on you repeatedly push you outside your coping capacity, leaving you feeling dysregulated, snappy, and wired but exhausted, or emotionally shut down.

Modern motherhood has become a somewhat impossible task. You're doing the work of an entire village but without a village. You're expected to be emotionally available 24/7, manage the household, run the family schedule, cook, clean, work, breastfeed, comfort, organize, anticipate everyone's needs, and maintain your relationships, all while functioning on sleep that wouldn't be considered humane in any other profession.

There's also the quiet expectation that you'll do it all cheerfully. That you won't lose your temper. That you'll enjoy the little moments. That you'll soak up the time because 'it goes so fast'. And, of course, those moments are precious, but that doesn't make the reality any less overwhelming.

What the science says

From a clinical perspective, this level of constant responsibility activates the stress-response system. Your cortisol rises. Your sleep becomes lighter. Your emotional threshold becomes narrower. Decision fatigue sets in. You become forgetful, irritable, tearful, anxious, or simply numb. Not because you're doing a bad job, but because you're doing too much.

I often compare motherhood to being the Wi-Fi router of the house. Everyone connects to you and everyone needs something from you, but when too many devices are connected at once, the system slows down. It's not broken; it's overloaded. The only difference is that routers don't feel guilty. Mothers do.

As mums, we are conditioned to believe you should be able to do it all and that asking for help means you're weak. That lowering your standards makes you lazy. That being overwhelmed means you're not cut out for this. The truth, however, is that you are not meant to run at full capacity every minute of every day. You are not built to absorb everyone's needs and ignore your own, and you are not meant to carry the mental load of an entire household without support.

There is nothing wrong with you. There is something hugely wrong with the expectations placed upon you. The moment you say, 'I can't do it all' is not the moment you fail – it's the moment you finally speak the truth and take control. What you need isn't more resilience. It's more support, more rest, and more room to just 'be'.

What you can do

- **Accept help:** This is one of the most powerful things a mother can do (and is also one of the hardest). We often associate help with weakness, when it's actually a sign of strength and wisdom. Humans are not designed to parent alone. Our nervous systems regulate themselves through connection. Sharing the load literally lowers cortisol and improves emotional resilience. Letting someone else take over a task is not an admission of failure. It is an act of self-preservation. Maybe that looks like:
  - letting your partner handle bedtime without micromanaging (see page 173 for my tips on stepping back)
  - accepting a meal from a neighbour

- hiring a cleaner every few weeks if you can
- sending your child to nursery even if you're at home
- saying yes when a friend offers to take your child for an hour
- using afterschool clubs
- allowing grandparents to help in their own way
- splitting tasks fairly with your partner (they are not 'helping', but sharing the load)
- asking other parents if you can car-share or swap pick-ups now and then
- if you're parenting alone, leaning on friends or family where possible, even for short breaks

It doesn't matter what the help looks like. What matters is that you don't carry everything alone.

- **Lower the bar (seriously):** I don't mean in a 'giving up' way, but in a compassionate and realistic way. Not every meal has to be home-made. Not every moment has to be magical. I promise you, your child does not need a Pinterest-worthy sensory tray every day. There will naturally be seasons of motherhood when survival is the goal. In those seasons, the floor might be messy, the meals might be basic, the laundry might live on the chair, and do you know what? That's OK. Your children will be fine. You will be fine. A lower standard doesn't mean a lower quality of parenting. It means you're protecting your energy. Your child needs you present, not perfect. Give yourself permission to do things the easy way:
  - buy the pre-chopped veg
  - say no to the thing that drains you
  - let someone else take over

  Because you don't need to be everything to everyone. 'Good-enough' parenting is safe, loving, and absolutely sufficient.

- **Take micro-breaks:** This tip changed everything for me.
  You don't need an hour-long bath or a spa day. You
  need a few minutes here and there to switch off your
  stress response. Sit in the car for a minute before going
  inside. Stand outside and feel the air on your face. Make a
  cup of tea and drink it *sitting down*. Hide in the loo for a
  60-second breathing reset. Your brain doesn't need long
  to switch from 'fight or flight' back into regulation. It just
  needs a moment. Block out pockets of time for yourself
  and treat them as non-negotiable.

'I'm Worried about Burnout'

We've seen how motherhood and stress often arrive hand in hand,
but we rarely talk about how quickly that stress can tip into
burnout. Burnout isn't just a buzzword for busy mums; maternal
burnout is a state of overwhelming mental, physical, and emotional
exhaustion caused by chronic parenting/juggling stress. It's what
happens when the demands placed on you continuously outweigh
the resources and support available to you, and it's something I've
also lived through. As a doctor, I thought I understood it enough
to avoid it, but when it happened to me, I didn't see it coming.

At the time, I was a full-time GP partner, carrying the
responsibility of running a practice, teaching medical students and
trainee doctors, and quietly pushing myself to keep up with my
male colleagues. At home, I had a young child and, like so many
high-achieving women, I was too proud to ask for help. Somewhere
deep down, I'd absorbed the idea that strength meant coping, and
that needing support meant I wasn't strong enough. I was also
trying to be a good friend, a present wife, a loving daughter, a
'fun' mum, and soon it all caught up with me.

When you're trying to give 100 per cent to everything, including
your social life, and still smiling through it all, it is easy for others
to miss how much you're actually carrying, but to borrow a phrase

from psychiatrist and bestselling author Bessel Van Der Kolk, my 'body kept the score'.[5] I was permanently exhausted but couldn't sleep. I felt numb and flat. I still showed up for my patients – that part of me stayed switched on – but I felt disconnected from myself. That experience humbled me. It changed how I practise as a doctor and how I show up in my own life.

Burnout in mothers isn't about being weak or dramatic – it's about being chronically overloaded in a world that expects women to carry everything with a smile. It's your body trying to get your attention because, the truth is, you weren't built to carry this alone.

This section is here to help you recognize the warning signs of burnout, understand why it's so common in modern motherhood, and, most importantly, begin finding your way back to yourself.

The signs of burnout

Burnout isn't the same as feeling tired or having a bad week. Burnout is deeper; you feel drained, detached, irritable, running on fumes, and unable to recharge even when you get a break. Clinically, burnout shows up as:

- emotional exhaustion
- feeling 'numb' or detached from parenting
- a sense of incompetence ('I'm failing at this')
- irritability, guilt, and overwhelm
- trouble concentrating
- changes in sleep and appetite
- a loss of joy in things you used to enjoy

And here's the scary bit: burnout doesn't just affect mothers, it affects the entire family system. When a mum is running on empty, it ripples outwards. Her patience thins, her energy drops, and her ability to stay emotionally present becomes harder. This isn't a reflection of her love or commitment – it's biology. As we've seen, when your nervous system is stuck in survival mode, your body prioritizes short-term coping over long-term connection. That means you might snap more easily, feel numb to joy, or struggle to tune in to your child's needs in the way you want to. And children, being the sensitive little barometers they are, pick up on that stress. They might become clingier, more anxious, or dysregulated themselves.

Burnout also affects relationships – with partners, friends, and even work colleagues. You can start to feel isolated, resentful, or disconnected, and the household dynamic can start to shift. But here's the hopeful bit: just as stress spreads, so does calm. When mums are supported to rest, to regulate, and to reconnect with themselves, the whole family benefits. That's why investing in maternal well-being isn't a luxury. It's a necessity – for everyone.

What the science says

Maternal burnout is far more common than people realize:[6]

- Research shows that up to 60 per cent of parents report feeling burnt out at some point, and mothers are significantly more likely to experience burnout than fathers. A 2022 meta-analysis found that one in four mothers meets the threshold for clinical levels of parental burnout.
- Burnout is closely linked to depression, anxiety, sleep problems, and chronic stress-related illnesses.
- Studies show that maternal burnout is associated with higher rates of emotional withdrawal, parental guilt, and, crucially, feeling unable to ask for help.

Researchers describe how prolonged stress in the parenting role can lead to emotional detachment, exhaustion, and a reduced sense of personal accomplishment, and is often accompanied by sleep disturbances, fatigue, mood changes, and reduced physical health.[7]

Why maternal burnout happens

Burnout isn't caused by one thing – it's the *accumulation* of many stressors and risk factors, including:

- **Sleep deprivation:** This is the biggest predictor of maternal mental health struggles. Broken or minimal sleep disrupts emotional regulation and reduces resilience, especially when it becomes chronic.
- **Feeding challenges:** This includes breastfeeding pain, latch issues, supply worries, and bottle-feeding guilt. Feeding your baby can become a source of physical pain, emotional stress, and deep self-doubt.
- **Birth trauma or difficult recovery:** As we saw in Chapter 1, a complicated or traumatic birth can leave lasting emotional scars, physical pain, and a sense of disempowerment that lingers well into the postnatal months – especially when healing is unsupported or dismissed.
- **Lack of support:** Partners working long hours, no family nearby, or feeling like you have to do it all alone increases stress and leaves mothers without anyone to lean on during tough moments.
- **High expectations:** Feeling pressure to parent 'perfectly' creates a constant sense of failure – as if anything short of superhuman is not good enough.
- **Mental load:** The constant invisible planning, remembering, anticipating, and organizing that mothers carry quietly in their heads creates cognitive and emotional exhaustion.
- **Comparison culture:** Social media, baby books, parenting forums, and well-meaning comments from others can create a relentless loop of 'shoulds' that erode confidence and increase self-doubt.

- **Juggling work and childcare:** Returning to work while managing childcare logistics, guilt, and competing demands can leave mothers feeling constantly torn and never fully present anywhere.
- **Caring for multiple children:** Meeting the needs of more than one child at different developmental stages multiplies the physical and emotional load, with little opportunity to rest or reset.
- **Financial stress:** Worries about income, childcare costs, reduced earnings, or job insecurity add a persistent background pressure that keeps the stress response switched on.
- **Perfectionism or high self-pressure:** Holding yourself to impossibly high standards means you're always falling short in your own eyes, even when you're doing your absolute best.
- **A baby with colic, reflux, or health issues:** Prolonged crying, frequent feeds, or medical worries increase sleep deprivation and anxiety, pushing parents into survival mode for long periods.

Many of these aren't under your control, which is why burnout isn't a sign of failure. It isn't a parenting flaw. It's a sign of a lack of support, rest, time, and recovery. It's a sign of being human. The good news is, it is reversible.

What you can do

- **Protect your sleep:** Sleep isn't a luxury – it's a biological need that protects your mood, memory, immune system, and emotional regulation. If you're in the trenches of newborn life, naps count. Share night duties with a partner or support person where possible, even just once or twice a week, and aim to go to bed earlier rather than 'staying up to get things done' – this trade-off rarely works in your favour. Prioritizing even short stretches of rest helps restore your emotional capacity.

- **Eat regularly:** Skipping meals or grabbing only caffeine and sugar can lead to unstable blood sugar, which makes mood swings, irritability, and energy crashes worse. Try to eat every three to four hours, and build meals around protein, fibre, and healthy fats – think wholegrain toast with nut butter, eggs with spinach, or yoghurt with seeds and berries. It doesn't have to be perfect, just regular and real. Adequate nourishment helps your brain and body cope with stress.

- **Stop comparing yourself to others:** Social media and parenting books can make it seem like everyone else has it all figured out – but that's not the reality. Every child is different. Every mum is different. Comparison often triggers feelings of shame or not being 'enough', which only adds to burnout. If you find yourself spiralling, unfollow, mute, or step back. Real life happens offline. Focus on what your child needs from *you*, not from someone else's highlight reel.

- **Talk before you hit a wall:** Please don't wait until you're in crisis to reach out. Talk to someone you trust or see your family doctor, health visitor, or perinatal mental health team early. There is so much they can do – from ruling out physical causes to exploring therapy, lifestyle support, medication, or (if appropriate) hormonal treatment. You don't need to struggle alone.

Punam's Prescription

Reclaim joy

Find small, realistic ways to reclaim a spark of joy – even in the busiest weeks. For example:

- take a brisk 10-minute walk with your favourite playlist
- light a candle and drink your tea while it's still hot
- watch something that makes you really laugh (yes, even a silly reel)
- sing at the top of your lungs in the car
- get under the duvet with a book and no guilt
- send a voice note to a friend who 'gets it'
- do your skincare routine slowly, like a ritual
- move your body just because it feels good
- journal your thoughts – even if it's messy
- say no to something and feel the relief
- have a solo coffee date with your favourite mug without any interruptions
- take yourself on a 'micro-adventure': a different route home, a new park, a random treat from the bakery
- sit outside for 5 minutes and notice the light, the sounds, and the breath in your chest

A wee tip: keep your own 'joy bank' in your phone Notes app. Add to it. Return to it. Pick one thing a day, even if it's just for 5 minutes. You deserve that.

Keep moving

Movement is one of the most effective treatments we have for stress, anxiety, and low mood. I'm not talking about gym sessions,

10k runs, or 'bouncing back'. I'm talking about incorporating gentle movement and stretching into your day to lower stress hormones, keep your mood stable, and reduce SNS activation.

The 10-minute reset walk

A brisk 10-minute walk can lift your mood for hours. Do it after nursery/school drop-off, during a lunch break, or with the buggy. Getting outside, especially in the morning light, is medicine for your nervous system. It helps regulate your sleep cycle, boosts mood, and lowers cortisol.

Kettle stretches

While the kettle boils, do:

- shoulder rolls
- gentle neck stretches
- calf stretches
- wrist rotations

Just 90 seconds of stretching signals to your brain: *I matter too.*

Dance therapy

Put on a favourite song and dance in the kitchen. It's an instant way to boost the mood and drop the cortisol, and your kids will love it too.

The 'choose one' rule

Each day, simply choose one of the following:

- move for 5 minutes
- stretch for 5 minutes
- breathe for 5 minutes

Consistency matters more than intensity.

Incorporate mindfulness tools

Mindfulness isn't about sitting in silence for 20 minutes or escaping to a retreat. If you had time for that, you probably wouldn't be reading this chapter. Mindfulness is simply the act of coming back into your body when your mind is racing or overwhelmed. When you're stressed, your nervous system needs these small anchor points.

Here are the tools that actually work in motherhood:

The four–two–six breath

This is my favourite mindfulness technique because it works quickly and anywhere – in the bathroom, in the car, even while feeding the baby. I often recommend it to mothers when I see them in clinic

Breathe in for four, hold for two, and breathe out for six. The longer exhale engages the PNS and helps bring down cortisol.

The 'name five things' reset

When your mind is spiralling, name:

- five things you can see
- four things you can touch
- three things you can hear
- two things you can smell
- one thing you can taste

This brings you straight back into the present moment. It's a great one to try with the kids too.

Mindfulness in motion

You don't need a quiet room; you need small awareness breaks:

- feel the warm water on your hands while washing up bottles

- notice your breath while rocking the baby
- ground your feet on the floor while pushing the buggy

These micro-moments genuinely regulate your nervous system.

The 'mini retreat' moment
- Step onto your doorstep or into the garden.
- Close your eyes for 10 seconds.
- Let the air hit your face.

This tiny sensory reset does more to lower your stress hormones than you'd think.

The 20-second body scan
Ask yourself: 'Are my shoulders tense? Is my jaw tight? Is my chest heavy?' Then soften one area at a time. When done regularly, this teaches your body to come out of fight-or-flight mode.

Use positive affirmations

Affirmations are not about pretending everything is fine. They're about interrupting the harsh inner critic that gets louder when you're overwhelmed. We know that compassionate self-talk can calm the nervous system, lower stress hormones, and improve emotional resilience.

Here are some affirmations that I've found genuinely help mums:

- **'I am doing enough':** Because you are – even when it doesn't feel like it.
- **'My feelings are valid':** Stress is stress. Sadness is sadness. You don't need a reason to be struggling. Every emotion you feel is valid and it matters.
- **'This moment will pass':** Nothing in motherhood is permanent – especially the hard bits.

- **'I deserve support:'** Needing help is not a failure; it's human.
- **'I am allowed to rest:'** Rest is medicine.
- **'Good enough is more than enough':** Decades of parenting research back this – children need presence, not perfection.[8]
- **'I am not alone':** Even when it feels like it, you're not.

Use these while in the shower, whisper them during a toddler meltdown, stick them on your fridge, or save one as your phone background. Little reminders like this can change the tone of your entire day.

Final Thoughts

If you're reading this chapter because you're overwhelmed or barely holding things together, please hear me: you will not feel like this forever.

Your brain is capable of healing. Your nervous system can recover. Your joy can return.

CHAPTER 9

'I Feel Isolated'

FINDING CONNECTION AGAIN

Motherhood is sold to us as a time of connection and, in many ways, it is. You grow a new human, your heart expands, and your family reshapes itself around this tiny person who needs you completely. But what we don't talk about nearly enough is how motherhood can also be one of the loneliest, most isolating periods of a woman's life. In fact, research shows that 72 per cent of mums feel invisible and 93 per cent feel unappreciated, unacknowledged, or unseen once they've had children.[1]

The isolation of motherhood is hard to explain to people who haven't felt it. It's not about being physically alone; in fact, you're rarely alone. You might have a baby attached to you, a toddler tugging at you, a school-aged child asking a thousand questions, or a teenager rolling their eyes at you, but the feeling of being on your own can sit under the surface. It can feel quiet, heavy, and private.

Isolation in motherhood can be down to lots of different things. It can be the isolation of making decisions constantly and silently, or carrying everyone's needs inside your mind all the time. It can be being touched all day, but not feeling truly seen or feeling guilty for struggling. It can be comparing yourself to other mums and assuming you're the only one finding it all so hard, even when you're trying your absolute best. In my clinic, mums often tell me that they feel lonely, and we know that loneliness is one of the strongest predictors of PND.[2]

From what I see in my GP role, mothers are more likely than any other group to feel disconnected from their communities. This isn't because we're doing anything wrong, it's because we're often mothering in a society that provides us with too little support and far too many expectations. Research shows that there are some countries that support mothers better than others though. For example, women in Sweden and Norway consistently rate the quality of maternal and newborn care higher than in other European countries, especially during the pandemic. Countries like Sweden, Finland, and the Netherlands also have more developed perinatal mental health programmes. In contrast, some low-resource countries have very limited postnatal care coverage.[3] These differences can really shape a mother's experience of support and connection.

Every week in my clinic, I see women trying to hold it all together. 'I love my baby, I really do,' they say. 'I just feel like I'm the only one not coping.' I've heard those words so many times – and I've lived them too. My first year of motherhood was one of the loneliest times of my life. I was recovering from a traumatic birth, navigating PND, and caring for a baby with severe reflux and feeding difficulties. Even though I had support around me, I often felt like I was quietly disappearing. It's a strange thing – to feel so full of love and yet so alone. What helped, in the end, was honesty. Speaking it out loud. Letting someone see the truth behind the smile. That's where the healing began.

This chapter is for you if you have ever felt like you're drowning in plain sight. If you've ever cried in the bathroom while everyone else in the house carried on as normal. If you've ever felt guilty for struggling when other mothers look like they're thriving. If you've ever wondered why you feel so disconnected from your partner, friends, or family when you're rarely on your own.

When to seek help

There are a few signs to watch out for that may indicate you would benefit from more support:

- **Loss of joy in daily interactions:** You're going through the motions, but not enjoying time with your children, partner, or yourself.
- **Avoiding social contact:** You're cancelling plans, withdrawing from WhatsApp groups, skipping baby groups, or avoiding the other mums at the school gates – even if you used to enjoy them.
- **Feeling invisible or forgotten:** You're expressing (or hinting at) thoughts like, 'No one checks in anymore' or 'I feel like I don't matter.'
- **Over-reliance on online validation:** You're regularly scrolling, comparing, or posting, but feeling worse afterwards – this is a sign you're seeking connection in the wrong places.
- **Disrupted sleep and appetite:** I don't mean the baby-related fatigue. Poor sleep or eating habits due to low mood, stress, or anxiety can be signs of emotional struggle.
- **Constant self-blame or harsh inner talk:** You're saying things to yourself like, 'I should be coping better' or 'Other mums are doing fine – what's wrong with me?'
- **Feeling overwhelmed by small tasks:** Daily chores or parenting duties feel impossible, triggering guilt or panic.
- **Increased irritability or numbness:** You're snapping at loved ones or feeling nothing at all: both can signal emotional burnout or disconnection.
- **Saying 'I'm fine', but looking depleted:** You're smiling on the outside while showing physical signs of exhaustion: dark circles, tearfulness, low energy, or lack of interest in self-care.

- **Lack of support system:** You don't have family nearby, partner support, or a close circle.

If any of these signs resonate with you, please reach out to a doctor, therapist, or support group. Seeking support is a strength, not a weakness.

'I Feel So Lonely'

One of the most helpful things I ever learnt – both as a GP and as a mum – is that loneliness in motherhood isn't just emotional. It's physiological; it's something your nervous system can feel long before your brain even finds the words.

During pregnancy, birth, and the early years, your nervous system undergoes one of the biggest transformations of your life. As we touched on in Chapter 8, the maternal brain becomes wired for hypervigilance – constantly scanning for danger, attuning to your baby's cues, and anticipating what might be needed next. This 'maternal vigilance' is a biological survival mechanism and it can lead to a feeling of disconnection from others.

When that isolation becomes chronic, it keeps the nervous system in 'threat mode', because humans need social contact to feel safe. Studies show that loneliness increases cortisol, reduces emotional regulation, affects sleep, and lowers resilience.[4] Your body interprets isolation as danger and, over time, that can make you feel on edge, drained, or even low. This is why so many mothers tell me they feel lonely even in a room full of people. It's because their nervous system is carrying everything silently and their mind is in survival mode.

Understanding this doesn't magically solve everything, but it does help soften the sense of shame or 'failurism' mothers often express. Your nervous system is doing what it was designed to do, but without the village it was designed to do it with.

The baby years: The most intense loneliness of all

This is the stage of motherhood that can feel the most paradoxical. You've never had less time to yourself and yet you've never felt more alone. You're needed all day, and sometimes all night, but the emotional connection can feel thin.

Newborn days often blur into each other. Feeding, nappy changes, rocking, pacing the house, trying to rest, trying to keep the house going, trying to manage relationships, trying to look like you're coping ... Weeks disappear before you realize you haven't had an adult conversation that wasn't about sleep or feeding or bowel movements. And because you're largely at home, especially if you're breastfeeding or recovering from birth, the world can feel very far away.

While maternity leave is a gift, it also often creates accidental isolation. So many women tell me they felt like they lost their identity in those early months. That going to a baby group felt overwhelming. That they felt guilty for not enjoying every moment. That they worried they were the only ones struggling. That everyone else seemed to be doing it right. Let me say this: you are not alone in that feeling. You're in the most profoundly demanding season of your life – emotionally, physically, and hormonally – and you're doing it without the societal support structures previous generations relied on. Newborn life is intense and isolating for many mothers, it's just we just don't see it or hear about it much because mothers have become experts at hiding it.

The school years: The isolation of invisible labour

Research has shown that loneliness was found to be highest in the preschool and school years, and that's no surprise to me as this stage comes with a whole new brand of isolation, the kind that comes from being the household project manager.[5] As we've discussed in previous chapters, you suddenly become the keeper of all the mental tabs: school trips, PE kits, permission slips, homework, reading logs, birthday parties, costumes, assemblies, clubs, packed lunches, playdates, dentist appointments, head lice outbreaks – all while working, cleaning, cooking, organizing, and maintaining relationships. It can feel relentless because the worst part is, it's invisible. No one sees how much you're doing – not your partner, not the school, not society – and so you feel secretly overwhelmed and quietly resentful. But because it's not 'hard' in the traditional sense, you don't feel allowed to talk about it. This is a huge source of maternal loneliness. You are working so hard, and no one sees it.

Also, because you're still wired for maternal vigilance, your nervous system is always scanning, 'Do we have the form? Did I reply to that email? Did I sign the reading book? When's the assembly? Did I say yes to that birthday party?' You're constantly managing tiny details, and it's that non-stop background noise that makes you feel isolated even when you're surrounded by people.

The teenage years: The loneliness of letting go

Mothers of teens often tell me that this is the most unexpectedly isolating stage. Not because the workload is highest, but because motherhood suddenly becomes quieter. It's much less hands-on, less visible, but, emotionally, it's far more complex.

Teenagers pull away for independence, which is healthy, but it can leave mothers feeling a bit redundant. And with that redundancy comes a grief and isolation that women rarely talk about. You miss the little hand in yours or being the centre of their world. You miss the certainty of routines, but, at the same time, you're trying to support them through exams, friendships, identity changes, hormones, first loves, first heartbreaks, risk-taking behaviours, and social pressures, and it feels like the stakes have never been higher.

The teenage years should come with a warning, for it is an emotional tightrope to try to: be present, but not intrusive; be encouraging, but not controlling; be supportive, but let them fall sometimes. This emotional balancing act can be deeply isolating.

If your teen is struggling, you may not want to share it with friends. You fear being judged or feel like you've failed somehow. You might lie awake worrying about their future while everyone else's lives appear to be moving smoothly. And if you're also juggling perimenopause – which many mothers of teens are – your own hormones can intensify that loneliness. Low oestrogen reduces your emotional resilience. Sleep is disrupted. Mood swings are common. Your brain feels foggy. Your libido drops. Your anxiety flares. You feel spread thin in every direction. It's the perfect storm for isolation, but the good news is that this stage also passes and there is support – you just need to know where to look for it.

What you can do

- **Reduce the noise:** Motherhood is overstimulating – the noise, the demands, the sensory overload – and it all ramps up your stress hormones. Turning down the intensity where possible creates space for connection. This might look like:
  - switching off notifications
  - limiting social media scrolling before bed
  - saying no to unnecessary obligations
  - creating tech-free evenings
  - lowering expectations around housework
  - Less noise = more space for connection.
- **Join or create a community in small ways:** You do not need to join 10 baby groups or force yourself into extroverted situations. Community can grow in quieter, gentler spaces:
  - a WhatsApp group for mums in your area
  - a library rhyme time or community event
  - a walking group
  - a coffee with one mum you trust
  - a parenting class

- an online support group
- a pelvic health physiotherapy course
- a mum-and-baby yoga session

Connection grows from small seeds.

- **Ask for help – without apology:** Accepting help isn't weakness, it's profound strength. It's how you build your village, feel less isolated, and protect your mental health.

'I Feel Like a Failure'

There is something uniquely tender about the way mothers speak when they feel like they're falling short. They soften their voice. They look down. They apologize before they even explain what's wrong. They use phrases like, 'I know I should be grateful' or 'Other mums have it harder.' And beneath those words is usually a deep fear that they aren't a good-enough mother. This feeling doesn't come out of nowhere. It's shaped by the world we live in. It shows up at baby groups, during chats at the school gates, in mother and toddler sessions, or even in WhatsApp groups full of milestone updates. It happens at every age and stage: when babies sit up, crawl, talk, walk, eat solids, sleep through; when kids start school, make friends, sit exams … You're constantly surrounded by glimpses of what other children are doing – and if yours is struggling, or you're finding it hard to cope, it can make you feel like you're the only one who hasn't got it figured out.

Social media – love it or hate it – can become both a lifeline and a trap when you're a mum. It keeps you connected, but it also gives you an endless reel of mothers who seem to be enjoying the stage that you're just trying to survive. You see the tidy houses, the matching outfits, the aesthetic buggies, the smiling selfies, the 'cosy newborn days', the toddlers who never throw pasta at the wall. These images are presented to us as normal, when, in reality, they are often edited, filtered, and selected from a hundred failed attempts. However, because mothers are often isolated and lacking real-life comparison, they assume social media is a mirror rather than a performance. I, too, fell for it when I was at my lowest mothering point.

I speak to so many women who tell me they feel guilty all the time – guilty for wanting a break, guilty for not enjoying the hard days, guilty for not breastfeeding, guilty for breastfeeding for 'too long', guilty for working, guilty for not working, guilty for shouting, guilty for allowing screens, guilty for shedding tears; basically, guilty for everything. Guilt becomes the background noise of motherhood and, when guilt sits inside you for long enough, it starts to sound like failure.

Society has for so long set standards that are unrealistic to achieve for the modern-day mother which, when unmet, lead to immense amounts of pressure and a sense of failure. It is exhausting. From the day you discover you are pregnant, there are expectations of what the 'perfect mother' would or should do, and nobody shies away from ensuring you know this. But here's the truth: almost every mother feels this way at some point. You are absolutely not failing. You are adjusting to a life-altering transition without the support you truly need.

What the science says

There's also a biological piece to feeling like a failure. In the weeks and months after birth, your hormones are moving in ways that affect your emotional resilience. Low oestrogen, disrupted sleep, nutrient depletion, chronic stress – all of these prime your brain for self-criticism. When you're tired and overwhelmed, you're far more likely to interpret small struggles as signs that something is wrong with you, rather than signs that you're just being human.

This 'not enoughness', no matter what you do, is draining and it is time for us to collectively acknowledge that mothers should never have had this expectation put upon them in the first place. We need to redefine motherhood. The 'perfect' mother, in my opinion, is the one who is present and authentic and human. She lets her kids see that she's trying her best and that she's showing up for herself, and for those she loves. In her imperfections, she is wonderfully perfect, and she is enough.

What you can do

- **Unfollow accounts that aren't serving you – and that includes in real life too:** Notice how you feel after spending time with certain people, whether online or in person. Do you feel heavier or lighter? Uplifted or drained? It's OK to set boundaries with the friends, groups, or digital spaces that chip away at your confidence. (See my Prescription on page 234 for my tips on having a digital detox.) Surround yourself with people who see and support you; the ones who don't expect perfection, who make space for the real conversations, and who remind you that you're doing better than you think.

- **Remember, the 'perfect' mother doesn't exist:** Embrace the chaos, let go of any perceived expectations and pressure to do everything and be everywhere, cooking and baking and crafting ... Do what you can, do what feels right, and remember your circumstances are different to everyone else's, so just do you. As a GP, I get to see what people's lives are like behind closed doors and I assure you, nobody has it spot-on.

- **Speak to mums of older kids:** This is something I often recommend to new mothers. There is something magical about being reassured by someone who has experienced the stage you're in. They've lived through the chaos and they remember how all-consuming it was, but they also carry a softness, a kind of hindsight that reminds you that nothing lasts forever. When they say, 'It gets easier' or 'You're doing brilliantly', it lands differently. It feels like wisdom, not pressure. These conversations remind you that you are not failing, you are simply in a tough season and seasons always change.

'I Feel Guilty That I Don't Have Time for My Partner Anymore'

We explored the physiological issues around not being in the mood for sex in Chapter 4, but let's also talk about how relationships change in the messy middle of raising children. Because they do change – even the strongest ones.

The shift from partners to co-parents is profound. You go from late-night conversations and spontaneous dinners to tag-teaming night feeds and sharing a calendar just to get some time alone. You're both sleep-deprived, overstimulated, and often just trying to get through the day. The roles you used to play in each other's lives – confidante, lover, friend – can quietly be replaced by logistics, handovers, and who's-doing-what. It's common to feel a quiet sadness that the ease you once had feels harder to reach.

So many mums internalize feelings of guilt when it comes to these shifts in their relationship. They worry they're letting their partner down. They worry their relationship is changing. They worry they're somehow responsible for the distance that appears when life becomes about nappies, school runs, and exhaustion. These are all such valid feelings.

Many mothers also tell me they miss being seen as more than 'Mum'. They miss the feeling of being desired, listened to, or held without someone else needing something from them. This isn't a sign that something is wrong with you or your relationship, it's a sign that you're in one of the toughest seasons. Relationships go through ebbs and flows, and parenthood brings some of the most intense waves.

It's important to acknowledge this and to name the change without blame because when we expect things to feel the same, we can start believing the worst: *Maybe we're not right for each other anymore*; *Maybe this is broken*; *Maybe I'm broken*. But sometimes, what's needed isn't an overhaul – it's just attention. Small acts of tenderness. Listening without solving. Making space to talk about more than the kids. Laughing again. Even just a moment to say: 'I miss us.'

That said, it's also important to recognize when things feel too hard; when there's a breakdown in communication, persistent resentment, emotional withdrawal, or a sense of being totally disconnected. If that's the case, please know that relationship counselling can be incredibly valuable. You don't have to be on the brink to benefit. Think of it like therapy for the team; a chance to understand each other again, rebuild safety, and find your way back to closeness. Relationships are living things, and they need tending, especially in the weeds of parenthood.

Remember: it's not a competition

Have you ever had an argument with your partner over who is more tired? In the early postpartum days, I would count the number of hours I slept versus my husband and lie there feeling resentful during the night while feeding the baby listening to his snoring – it felt so unfair. It's no wonder that sleep deprivation was once used as a form of torture because it really does distort your entire way of being – it impacts the way you think and feel, and leaves you feeling desperate at times.

Resentment towards a partner is a common phenomenon and a very valid experience, especially among new mums. This is a feeling that results from several different factors including the obvious sleep deprivation, but also hormonal influences and inequities in childcare responsibilities (remember, mums take on over twice as many daily jobs as dads)[6] which give rise to feelings of frustration and a psychological disconnection from your partner.

The same is felt when partners appear to have more personal time compared to the mother, who is relied upon more heavily by the baby. In fact, this is backed up by research, which has shown that men (in the UK) enjoy nearly five more hours of leisure time per week than women.[7]

As tempting as it may be to give your partner the silent treatment, moan about them to a friend, or simply have a cathartic rant, these will never solve the issue. Instead, have an open conversation with them and share your feelings because they might not even be aware that there is even an issue.

What you can do

- **Have open, honest conversations:** Express your concerns and, if you feel overloaded and therefore resentful, share out responsibilities and create a timetable. Don't feel ashamed about admitting that you feel disconnected and that you need help.
- **Rekindle connection:** You don't need elaborate date nights every week. Instead, you can rekindle connection with your partner by:
  - watching a show together
  - sitting for 10 minutes after the kids' bedtime to check in
  - going for a walk together
  - sharing one task
  - being honest without blame

  Connection doesn't have to be glamorous, it just has to be intentional.

'I Don't Feel I Have Anything in Common with My Friends Anymore'

Trying to understand and accept the way friendships shift is one of the quiet griefs of motherhood. It's rarely talked about, but nearly every mother feels it in some form.

Motherhood changes you. Of course it does. It changes your priorities. It changes how you spend your time, what you worry about, how tired you are, and how available you are – and sometimes your friendships don't change at the same pace. Friends without children might not understand why you cancel plans, why you're tired all the time, or why you're not as present or 'fun' as you once were. Friends with children might be in a different rhythm or facing their own struggles. This can lead to feeling disconnected from people you once felt deeply close to, and that can really hurt.

This is part of the motherhood health penalty too. For many women, social circles quietly shrink after having a child – not because they've done anything wrong, but because time, energy, and availability fundamentally change. Research suggests that around 80 per cent of young mothers report meeting friends less often after having a baby, which helps explain why this sense of loss and disconnection is so common.[8] Once your child is at school, the playground can feel like a strange form of social politics and if you're already stretched thin, navigating that space can feel lonely too. Some school mums become wonderful allies while others might stay on the surface.

Some friendships will grow with you. Some will pause and return years later. Some will shift into something gentler. Some might naturally fade. This doesn't mean you've done something wrong. It means that life has changed and, yes, you have changed. We seem to view change as a negative transition when, in actual fact, you are simply growing into your next season and that's OK.

New friendships often emerge in motherhood too, so it's not all doom and gloom. There will be the woman you meet at playgroup, the mum at the school gate who smiles at you knowingly, or the colleague who whispers, 'Me too'. These friendships are not there to replace old ones, but they expand your emotional support network for the season you're in.

What you can do

- **Communicate honestly:** If you feel you're losing touch with friends, one of the kindest things you can do for yourself is to be honest. Saying something like, 'I'm overwhelmed, I love you, I just don't have the capacity right now,' can save a friendship. People don't need perfect communication, they just need to understand where you're at.

- **Reintroduce 'micro-connections':** When your capacity is low, long conversations feel impossible, but tiny touches of connection – a 30-second voice note, a photo, a meme, or a quick 'thinking of you' message – still count. These micro-moments keep friendships alive. Connection doesn't always mean big gestures or huge changes. Sometimes it begins with tiny shifts that help your nervous system feel safer and less alone.

Punam's Prescription

Have a digital detox

Protect your mind by switching off notifications, setting app limits, and unfollowing pages that make you feel inadequate. Social media can feel like both a lifeline and a landmine. It connects us, especially in the isolating trenches of motherhood, but it also bombards us with noise, comparisons, unrealistic expectations, and information overload. Every scroll chips away at your focus, your mood, and, crucially, your sense of self. That's not a personal weakness – it's neuroscience.

Constant digital input overstimulates your brain, keeps your nervous system on high alert, and reduces your ability to concentrate or regulate emotions. Even 10-minute scrolls here and there add up across the day, draining the very bandwidth you're trying to protect. So, start small:

- Mute or unfollow accounts that leave you feeling less-than.
- Set phone-free times: during meals, bedtime, or the first 30 minutes after waking.
- Try one notification-free evening a week.
- Swap one scroll for something that nourishes you: a short walk, a chat with a friend, even just sitting in silence.

Protect your mental space like it's a precious resource, because it is. Your brain was not designed to absorb the constant noise of 24/7 input. Stillness isn't a luxury, it's medicine for your mind.

Schedule regular family time

I recommend choosing a day at the weekend that is a strict, non-negotiable family day. I realized post-lockdown how precious this was for me to feel less alone as a mother but also for us all as a family. We chose Saturdays (unless something important comes up) as our non-negotiable family day. This could be a day of lazing around the house, going for a walk together or out for a meal, or a day trip/experience.

A family unit is also a team and it can be helpful to hold a family meeting once a month, once a fortnight, or every Sunday (I personally find this a great day to do it) to sit with the calendar and chat about roles and responsibilities for every member over the coming week or month. This could include meal planning, tasks, and chores, as well as fun activities. School-age kids can take on small responsibilities, teens can contribute more meaningfully, and even toddlers can help in tiny ways. I find kids enjoy being part of this as it gives them some control.

Involving your kids like this can reduce your mental load which, in turn, can help you reconnect and reduce any feelings of isolation. It also teaches them resilience, belonging, and responsibility.

Name your feelings out loud

When you keep everything bottled up, shame grows in the silence. But when you name your feelings – even if it's just quietly, even if it's just once – something powerful happens: you break that silence. You create a crack for light to come through.

Try this: take a breath and say aloud, 'I feel overwhelmed'; 'I feel like I'm failing'; or 'I feel disconnected from myself.' There is no shame in this. These are human experiences, not personal flaws. You don't have to carry these feelings alone. Tell someone you trust, whether that's your partner, your best friend, your sister, or your family doctor. You don't need to have all the words. You just need to start.

- Saying, 'I feel lonely' is not a failure: it's the beginning of support.

- Saying, 'I'm not coping' is not a sign of weakness: it's the first step towards feeling better.
- Saying, 'I'm not myself' doesn't mean you've lost who you are: it means you're ready to find her again, with help.

You are not a burden. Your feelings matter. And support exists, but it often starts with that brave moment of honesty. You have got this!

Practise self-compassion

So many mums speak to themselves in ways they would never speak to another person, but that critical inner voice simply fuels isolation. It's so important, therefore, to bring more self-compassion into your daily life. Here are some simple ways to do just that:

The friend test

If you wouldn't say it to a friend you adore, don't say it to yourself. This sounds simple, but it takes practice. Many of us have spent years – decades, even – with a harsh inner voice that jumps straight to criticism. Rewiring that voice doesn't happen overnight, but it is possible. The trick is to notice it first.

Catch the moment you speak to yourself in a way you never would to someone you love. Pause. Then rewrite that thought in a kinder voice – not fake positivity, but gentle, honest compassion. This is where affirmations come in again, to offer your nervous system an anchor – a more supportive voice when your internal dialogue is spiralling. And the more you do it, the more you train your brain and body to accept this kindness. Over time, you build your emotional muscle and you become more resilient, not because everything feels good, but because you know how to hold yourself when it doesn't.

Try these reframes when you catch yourself in a spiral:

- **When you feel overwhelmed:** 'I am doing my best with the resources I have.'
- **When you feel like your body is failing or changed:** 'My body is capable of incredible things.'
- **When you're just having a bad day:** 'It's OK to feel sad/ bad/alone – this moment will pass.'

Then lean into something that soothes you – a walk, a favourite uplifting show, a good cry, or a phone call with a friend. Give yourself full permission to have low days without making them mean anything about your worth.

Compassionate self-talk is one of the most powerful tools you can use to ride the ups and downs of motherhood without losing yourself.

Hand-on-heart pause

Place your hand gently on your chest and say: 'Of course I'm finding this hard. Anyone would.' This activates oxytocin, which is the body's love and bonding hormone, and immediately softens your stress response.

Little permission slips

Write yourself one each morning:

- Today I'm allowed to rest.
- Today I'm allowed to ask for help.
- Today I'm allowed to not be perfect.

Small acts of self-kindnesses change how you feel you are coping.

Break the 'superwoman' script

Swap 'I should ...' for 'I could ...' It reduces pressure and gives back control.

Celebrate micro-wins
I'm not talking about the big achievements, but the tiny ones:

- you drank water
- you ate a proper meal
- you took a breath before reacting
- you got through the day

These are victories. These matter. And they will reduce the feeling that you are somehow failing.

Final Thoughts

Feeling isolated doesn't mean you're ungrateful or doing anything wrong; it means you're human and in a season that stretches every part of you. The truth is, you were never meant to carry all of this alone. You deserve support, compassion, rest, and connection just as much as the people you care for every day. Even on the days when you feel invisible or disconnected or unsure of who you're becoming, please remember this: you are still here, still showing up, still loving with everything you have. That is not isolation. That is resilience.

Slowly, gently, and with the right support and the right people around you, you will feel connected again, both to others and to yourself.

CHAPTER 10

'There's No Time for Me'

HEALING, REBUILDING, AND PROTECTING YOUR FUTURE HEALTH

As a mum, you often put yourself last, and it's not because you don't care – it's because you care so much. You feed everyone else, remember every birthday and occasion, celebrate everyone's wins, show up for as many school events as possible (even when they are scheduled for the middle of the working day!), and look after everyone when they're poorly. Then, by the end of the day, you collapse in front of the telly or in bed with your phone, mindlessly scrolling and questioning why you have no more left to give. The battery quickly loses charge, and you have none left for you.

Many parents feel selfish taking time out to care for themselves, but looking after yourself is so important. When you are well, your whole family benefits. That's not indulgence – that's essential maintenance. The cost of not prioritizing self-care is a measurable, medical health penalty – one that builds quietly and slowly over time. I see so many mothers experience this phenomenon – and the science backs it up (see box below).

What the science says

There's good evidence showing that chronic parental stress and burnout are linked to measurable physical and mental health penalties over time.[1] Large reviews of the research consistently find that higher parental stress is associated with lower overall well-being: including fatigue, poor quality of life, and reductions in psychological and physical functioning. A recent meta-analysis of more than 22,000 parents found a significant negative association between parental stress and general well-being, meaning that as stress increases, happiness, life satisfaction, and physical and emotional health decrease.

Let's be honest, nobody warns you about how little time you will have for yourself once you have kids. Even personally, I knew it would be challenging to find the time to be as present in my social life as I once was, but I had no idea that my social interactions would become the least of my worries – I struggled to even find time for simple, personal self-care after the birth of my firstborn. In my former, non-mother life, I wouldn't have been seen dead out of the house with no make-up on, so when I found myself in the supermarket with my PJs as a base layer, not having brushed my teeth or showered, it was a real low. This is often what life as a new mother, especially a mother with little external support, can look like though. Apart from my husband who worked full-time, I had little family and friend support around me. It was me, myself, and I – and my little baby with severe silent reflux – trying to get through every day and, with the endless feeding/posseting/changing cycles, I was exhausted. Even when I did find small pockets of time for me, I had no energy to do anything with them.

It can be a strange and disorienting feeling when basic tasks – like brushing your teeth or having a shower – start to feel impossible. Especially when, not long ago, you were someone who could juggle work, home, and life with confidence. I remember questioning myself constantly: 'You're a doctor, Punam. You look after people every day – how are you not able to look after yourself?' The sense of inadequacy and failure was all-encompassing.

The reality, however, is that the minute we become mothers, we fall to the bottom of the priority list. It's almost a reflex. You treat your baby's nappy rash like a medical emergency, but your own eczema flare-up? 'Ah, it'll settle.' You make sure your child eats colourful, balanced meals, lovingly prepared snacks, and maybe even a probiotic added in because you've swotted up on the benefits. You, however, settle for leftovers consumed standing up and as quickly as possible. Sound familiar?

From the early days of using baby wipes to 'cleanse' your skin to the quiet exhaustion of midlife, your body carries the weight of everything you have poured out. This isn't about guilt, it's about recognition; something I have seen in my elders – my grandmothers, aunts, and mother – and something I hear daily from the incredible women I see every day as a GP. Here's the truth – and I say this with all the love and understanding in the world: you can't run on scraps for long. And not without consequences. Putting yourself last doesn't make you a better mum. It just makes you a tired, depleted one. And, over time, it chips away at your health. However, the good news is you can reclaim your healthcare needs and that doesn't have to mean adding to the already intense mother load.

This chapter is dedicated to every mother who has ever said, 'I feel like I just don't have time for me.' We are going to unpack what's happening beneath the surface and I'll show you some small, practical, evidence-based steps to start reclaiming your time for your health across every phase of motherhood. I will help you create small, clinical wins that fit into your reality and not some unattainable wellness plan – because, let's be honest, who has got time for that?

'The Baby Needs Everything ... But What About Me?': The First Two Years

This is the chapter of motherhood when your body has undergone something seismic and yet, everyone moves on as if nothing has happened as all the focus instantly shifts to the baby. You get signed off at a vague 'six-week check' (if you're lucky) and then it's on to the full-time job of feeding, soothing, and surviving. During this time, you are likely under-slept, underfed, and under-acknowledged. Women often mask how depleted they are by pushing through and keeping busy. They smile and say they're fine, even when they're running on fumes. Many wear make-up to hide tiredness, rely on caffeine to get through the day, and minimize their symptoms, brushing off things like pain, fatigue, or low mood. They cancel their own appointments, miss meals, skip rest, and delay seeking help because the baby's needs always come first. And because so many mums around them are doing the same, it can feel normal – even expected – to quietly struggle.

One mum told me that after her baby arrived, everyone was so focused on the newborn that she felt like she'd disappeared. She was breastfeeding round the clock, barely sleeping, and living on cereal and cold tea, yet every conversation started with, 'How's the baby?' Her own needs felt invisible. She described feeling off in ways she couldn't quite explain: her hair was thinning, her skin looked dull, she felt bloated, foggy, and constantly on edge. She wasn't unwell in the traditional sense, but she wasn't well either. This phase – from birth to toddlerhood – is when women are at peak risk of being physically depleted and, more importantly, clinically invisible. It's therefore vital that we are listened to and given the space to heal so we can protect our future health.

Let's look at what is going on in your body during these early years and uncover some tips to reclaim some time for you.

Your skin

As we've explored, after birth, the hormones that had been giving you that beautiful pregnancy glow instantly go into freefall. Oestrogen and progesterone, which were high during pregnancy, drop dramatically in the first few days postpartum. If you are breastfeeding, oestrogen levels stay lower for longer. When oestrogen levels drop, it results in lower collagen, which is an essential building block for good hair, nails, and skin. Alongside this, your cortisol levels – this is your stress hormone – start to climb and stay high thanks to broken sleep, feeding demands, new mum anxiety, and emotional overwhelm. So, what does this do to your skin?

- increased dryness and sensitivity
- flare-ups of pre-existing conditions like eczema, dermatitis, rosacea, acne, and psoriasis
- puffiness or darkness under and around the eyes: hormonal shifts make blood vessels under the eyes more visible and fatigue slows down circulation and lymphatic drainage, contributing to puffiness
- melasma (also called 'chloasma' or 'pregnancy mask', where brown or greyish patches of pigmentation develop, usually on the face) can linger from pregnancy and can be worsened by sun exposure and inflammation
- thinner skin that looks duller as a result of lower collagen

We underestimate how much our skin reflects what's happening on a cellular level in our bodies – the hormonal chaos, sleep deprivation, and nutritional depletion all take their toll. Higher cortisol levels mean more inflammation on a deeper, cellular level too, which delays healing during skin flare-ups. Alongside this, during this period, we are at risk of being nutritionally depleted and therefore lower levels of essential skin vitamins and minerals like iron, B12, and zinc cause slower skin regeneration (see page 43 for more on the symptoms of vitamin and nutrient deficiencies).

It's easy to see why the skin doesn't 'skin' as well as it should in new mothers. Incidentally, this is a similar phenomenon during perimenopause where, again, our oestrogen levels begin to drop (more on this in a bit). So, what can help?

Forget those Instagram mums touting their 'quick fixes' and stick to a simple, realistic skincare routine that works for *your* skin – all you really need is a gentle cleanser for your skin type, a moisturizer, and a daily SPF. That's it. (See my Prescription on page 264 for the ingredients to look out for.) Don't get sucked into the products marketed at 'new mums' with a promise to help boost your skin that will likely cost you an arm and a leg. The truth is, nothing can replace a healthier, balanced lifestyle, which is where the deficiencies are stemming from.

When it comes to skin, it isn't about vanity, it's about vitality. Your skin is always talking to you, so pay attention and nourish it.

Nutrition

It's so interesting how our 'eating for two' mentality quickly disappears after the baby is born, when you find yourself eating toast crusts and washing it down with cold tea. (Don't worry, I've been there too, so there's no judgement from me here.) It's hard finding the time or energy to cook for yourself when you have a new baby or toddler in tow – and all the demands that come with that. I get it, but I do feel we've normalized this new mum lifestyle. We need more education around why this shouldn't be the norm and how damaging it can be to maternal health – and that's what I'm here for.

Mothers' bodies actually need more nutrients after birth than during pregnancy, particularly if they are breastfeeding. Producing breast milk requires extra energy and draws on the body's stores of key nutrients like protein, calcium, iodine, and vitamin A, to name a few. On top of that, the postnatal body is healing – from tissue repair to rebuilding iron stores lost during birth – all of which increases nutritional needs. Yet most women receive far less support and guidance on their diet after birth than they do during pregnancy. This matters, because poor nutrition in the early postpartum period can impact a mother's energy, immune system, mood, and long-term health. If you're feeling depleted, low, or run-down, this could be part of the reason, and it's absolutely something worth addressing.

What's more, your digestive system goes through changes postnatally too. Hormonal shifts can slow down gut motility, especially in the first few weeks after birth. Many new mums experience bloating, constipation, or sluggish digestion – often made worse by dehydration, iron supplements, or just not eating regularly. And let's not forget the fear of that first poo post-birth (yes, it's a thing!). If you're not eating enough fibre, drinking enough water, or fuelling your body with the right nutrients, your gut health takes a hit – which in turn affects your energy, skin, mood, immunity, and overall recovery. Your gut really is your second brain, and it needs just as much care as every other part of you during this stage.

A lot of people talk about food as fuel which it is, especially in those early years of motherhood. However, postnatal nutrition isn't just about energy – it's about repair, regulation of systems, and long-term resilience. Your body has done something *huge*. It has lost blood, broken down tissue, shifted organs about, and grown a new human. And yet, society has normalized mums skipping meals, surviving on caffeine, and feeling wiped out – that's just how 'hashtag mum life' rolls, right? Wrong. Good nutrition isn't a luxury during this season, it is medicine.

What the science says

Here's why postnatal nutrition matters:

1. **Tissue healing:** Whether you had a vaginal delivery or a C-section, your body needs extra protein, vitamin C, zinc, and iron to rebuild muscle, skin, and connective tissue.
2. **Hormone regulation:** Your thyroid and adrenal glands have

to adapt fast to the changes your body is going through and, for this, they need adequate amounts of iodine, selenium, B vitamins, and magnesium to keep your metabolism stable.

3. **Mood and brain health:** The drop in oestrogen plus the sleep deprivation affect neurotransmitters like serotonin and dopamine. Nutrients like omega-3, iron, and vitamins B6 and B12 are vital for keeping these stable.

4. **Milk production if breastfeeding:** You need around 500 extra calories per day if making milk and this also requires higher levels of iodine, calcium, vitamin A, and essential fatty acids.

5. **Bone and muscle recovery:** You lose bone mineral density and muscle mass quite quickly postnatally, which is reversible with good nutrition to replace the calcium, protein, and vitamin D.

I know how challenging it can be to make time to cook from scratch for yourself daily when you are in the thick of it, so here are some simple ideas on how to build it in without the faff:

Breakfast ideas
- porridge + chia seeds + almond or peanut butter (add in some berries for extra vitamins)
- Greek yoghurt + berries + granola
- boiled eggs + wholegrain or sourdough bread (top with some avocado for extra goodness)

Quick lunch ideas
- batch-cooked lentil, vegetable, or chicken soup (or buy tinned if it's easier) + sourdough bread
- tuna wrap + grated cheese or salad
- hummus + oatcakes + cherry tomatoes + boiled egg

'Mum snacks'
- a handful of nuts
- a square of dark chocolate
- apple slices + peanut butter
- full-fat yoghurt + some seeds on top

I always have these kinds of snack with me at work or in the car so the kids and I can pick at them.

For those extra time-poor days
- blitz a 'whatever's in the fruit/veg basket' smoothie and freeze it so you can grab it on those days when things just feel too difficult
- buy pre-chopped everything to save you time and energy when you're really up against it
- use frozen everything: spinach, peas, berries … you get the gist
- tinned fish is always great for those fast-hitting omega-3s (think mackerel, sardines, and tuna)

These are just some super simple things I do. Like most mums, I don't have much time, but I never want to let that get in the way of my nutritional needs – and I want to empower you to do the same.

When to seek help

If you are constantly tired, foggy, feeling low, achey, or your hair is thinning despite eating well, check in with your doctor to get your full blood count, ferritin (iron stores), zinc, B12, folate, vitamin D, and thyroid tests done.

Note: It is very normal to go through a hair-shedding phase after birth; however, if this persists or is worsening, please get it checked.

Postnatal movement

When it comes to movement postnatally, it's not about 'getting your pre-baby body back' or weight loss. It's about healing, rebuilding, and protecting your future health as a mother who wants to be there with her children, growing and thriving alongside them, stronger than ever before. However, the reality is where do we find the time? I hear you!

With the 24/7 shifts of new mum life – the constant feeding, bleeding, pain, leaking, and healing – exercise is often the *last* thing on your mind or your to-do list. Without guided, purposeful recovery, though, the risk of long-term problems rises dramatically and this is something I wish more women were informed about antenatally:

- Pelvic floor dysfunction is present in one in three women postpartum, often worsened by delayed or no rehabilitation.[2]
- Muscle mass loss accelerates without resistance training and is vital for women to pay attention to as muscle is protective for metabolism, posture, and mood.
- Postnatal women are at an increased risk of lower back pain, urinary incontinence, prolapse, core instability, and joint laxity due to the lingering effects of the hormone relaxin that spikes during pregnancy.

Please remember this is not me telling you to do anything you don't feel like doing. This is simply me – as your GP best friend – helping to educate you on the consequences of no movement later down the line.

What the science says

The weeks and months after birth are a unique period of recovery and recalibration for the entire body. Hormones are shifting, tissues are healing, and the body is trying to return to its pre-pregnancy state while also adapting to the demands of new motherhood (like lifting, feeding, broken sleep, and stress). If movement is completely avoided during this time, the body can start to 'set' into dysfunctional patterns, such as poor posture, weakened core, and weakened pelvic floor muscles, which become harder to reverse later. When movement is completely absent or avoided:

- postural dysfunction becomes a way of life: think rounded shoulders, a curved spine, and a forward tilt to the pelvis
- core muscles remain weak, creating ongoing back and pelvic pain
- the pelvic floor remains weak, resulting in increased risks of leaking, heaviness, and prolapse
- fatigue worsens due to reduced circulation and endorphin production
- long-term heart and metabolic health is neglected

In short, this isn't about 'bouncing back' – it's about laying the foundations for your future health.

Incorporating movement can be a particular issue for women from Black and ethnic minority backgrounds where the culture advocates full bed rest for several weeks after birth. While I love this element of prioritizing rest, intentional movement needs to feature as an integral part of the healing process. I know this personally as someone from an Indian heritage – we have a brilliant culture of resting and feeding mamas, but we do not encourage movement and, as we've seen, this can have long-term consequences.

Doable movement for exhausted mums
Firstly, it's important to start slow and wait until you feel ready (around four to six weeks postnatal is a good time) and after

medical clearance if you have had any complications. If you have had a C-section, you may need to wait a little longer. However, remember, pelvic floor rehabilitation must start from day one (see page 90 for some guidance on this).

Begin with:

- **Breathing and pelvic floor activation:** Breathe from the rib cage with a slow squeeze as if you are holding your pee mid-flow, and then release.
- **Gentle core rehabilitation:** Try heel slides, glute bridges, and wall sits. (You can find guidance online to ensure you do these safely and effectively.)
- **Walking:** Even 5 to 10 minutes a day improves mood, sleep, and insulin sensitivity by helping your body use blood sugar more effectively. Try buggy walks – I loved these when my two were little; it's such an easy but low-impact cardio workout.
- **Stretching:** However you fancy it, stretch your body.

These take no time at all and you can easily weave them into your day no matter how tired you feel. The goal should be at least 10 to 15 minutes of movement per day across three to four days per week with *zero* pressure to 'bounce back'. And remember, your pelvic health physiotherapist is your best friend (see page 73 for more information on how they can help).

What you can do

- **Stay hydrated:** Current guidelines in the UK are to aim to drink six to eight cups or glasses of fluid a day, or enough so that your pee is a clear pale-yellow colour.
- **Eat to support your skin:** Your skin eats what you eat, so make sure it's the good stuff!
  - Make your baby or toddler's plate and copy it for yourself, adding in extra protein and upping your

portion size – your body needs it. Some easy ways to boost your protein include: stir in nut butter, add a boiled egg, sprinkle on hemp or chia seeds, mix in Greek yoghurt, or include cooked chicken, tinned lentils, or cottage cheese.

- ○ Add one plant-based source of iron per day (any greens, beans, or seeds).
- ○ Boost your calcium with a glass of milk, some tofu, cheese, or a yoghurt.
- ○ Use tinned oily fish two to three times a week – it counts.
- ○ Keep those 'mum snacks' handy – in your handbag or in the car.
- ○ If you need a multivitamin to support this, that's OK, as long as it's not instead of eating well.
- ○ Take a daily vitamin D supplement (10mcg in the UK). This supports bone health, muscle function, immunity, and helps your body absorb calcium more effectively – this is especially important for mums who are indoors a lot or breastfeeding. Get your iron, zinc, and vitamin D levels checked if your skin is really dull or flaky.

- **Seek support:** Get help if you can so you can get some rest and learn to say no to protect your own energy and needs.

'I've Got a Bit More Space Now … But Still No Energy!': The Preschool/School Years

Your little one is now in preschool or school and you might – finally – have some pockets of time. Maybe you're back at work or exercising regularly and yet, your body still feels like it's running on empty. It could be that those initial years of physical depletion are starting to surface. The skipped meals, interrupted sleep, and lack of core or pelvic recovery can all show up in this phase – in your energy levels, your posture, your skin, your joints, and your mood. But, even with the kids at school for around six and a half hours a day, you are still giving more than you are replenishing. The snacks, drinks, and book bags get packed, the children eat breakfast, and you rush out the door with a half-drunk cup of coffee (the second of the morning) – the to-do list is never-ending. The pressure may seem lighter, but, as we've seen, it is hard to juggle it all and it can really take its toll.

Many women in this phase share their frustrations with me in clinic – 'I should be feeling more like myself now' – but the truth is, your body is still in repair mode. The good news is it's not too late and, with support, you can avoid long-term symptoms from creeping in.

What the science says

Cortisol levels usually remain high in this phase, especially with the modern-day 24/7 lifestyles we lead which, combined with the last few years of broken sleep and overdoing it, all catch up. These elevated cortisol levels can lead to more insulin resistance, leaving you craving those sweet treats, followed by energy crashes and hunger pangs after eating – and the cycle continues.

Diets low in fibre and high in ultra-processed convenience foods can reduce gut microbial diversity, and research shows this matters beyond digestion.[3] Fibre feeds the beneficial bacteria in your gut, which, in turn, produce metabolites that support immune function, inflammation control, and metabolic health. When dietary fibre is low, the composition of the gut microbiome shifts unfavourably, a state known as 'dysbiosis', which has been linked to inflammation and wider health issues. Ultra-processed foods and diets high in refined sugars and saturated fats are strongly associated with microbial imbalance and disruption of the gut barrier. Changes in the microbiome are now being connected to mental health, immune regulation, and even interactions with hormone pathways, including those that influence serotonin, inflammation, and metabolic function. All of this gives us a clue as to why poor diet and low fibre are linked with symptoms like anxiety, low mood, bloating, and fatigue – the gut and brain are communicating constantly.

Something I see a lot in women in my clinic and in my own group of friends and family is that we don't take fibre or our gut health seriously, and they're much more important than we have been taught as kids.

Nutrition

This season is very important because you're in a window where nutrition has the power to radically change your mood, gut, and hormonal resilience. Try to focus on:

- **Protein:** This is vital for muscle maintenance and hormonal balancing. Think chicken, eggs, yoghurt, lentils, nuts, tofu, and cheese.
- **Fibre:** This is critical for gut health, stable energy, and blood sugar. Good sources include oats, veg, fruit with their skins on, legumes, and seeds.
- **Healthy fats:** These are vital for brain and hormone support and can be found in oily fish, avocados, seeds, olive oil, and full-fat dairy.
- **Calcium and vitamin D:** These are needed for bone strength. Milk, fortified plant milks, green veg, and tinned fish are all good sources.
- **Magnesium:** This is lesser known but so important for mood, sleep, and blood sugar control. Magnesium can be found in dark chocolate, bananas, spinach, and almonds.

When to seek help

Many women don't realize their health is lagging until it starts to impact daily life. Symptoms that need a doctor's review include:

- worsening fatigue
- irregular or heavier periods
- brain fog or low mood
- bloating, constipation, or pain
- skin changes or hair loss
- persistent pelvic discomfort
- unintentional weight loss

Ask for a blood test including a full blood count, iron, ferritin, B12, folate, vitamin D, thyroid, urine dip, and a physical examination with your blood pressure and body mass index (BMI).

Restorative movement

It's so important to reframe movement during this phase because while you're likely running around after the kids, your movements are all reactive, not restorative. They do count, but not in the long-term meaningful way we need them to. As we explored in Chapter 5, when we are constantly carrying our 12+kg toddlers about, these kinds of repetitive and asymmetrical movements in fact strain the joints, back, and pelvic floor. If your core and glutes are still weak from pregnancy, the load goes through to the lower back. Most women around this stage haven't returned to regular strength work yet and this runs the risk of progressive muscle loss.

If you are time-poor, start slow:

- **Ten minutes a day of bodyweight moves:** Think squats, wall push-ups, and glute bridges. Get your tots involved and make it fun.
- **Stretching:** This will help to counter those years of baby-carrying posture – your shoulders, neck, back, and hips will thank you.
- **Walking:** Aim for a brisk 30-minute walk most days – even if it's broken into chunks of 10 minutes, during lunch breaks, drop-offs, and pick-ups; it all counts.
- **Balance work:** Stand on one foot while brushing your teeth and alternate – it's so easy and it helps to strengthen your core, glutes, and stabilizing muscles around your ankles and hips. It also improves your coordination and proprioception (your body's awareness of where it is in space), which can help prevent falls and injuries – this is especially important for mums carrying children or multitasking on the go.

These are all free, can be done in your own time, anywhere, and require nothing but a commitment to yourself.

What you can do

- **Prevent energy crashes:** Try to include a source of protein (like eggs, beans, yoghurt, cheese, chicken, fish, or nuts) and some fibre (like wholegrains, fruit, veg, or legumes) in every meal or snack. This helps stabilize your blood sugar, which in turn supports better mood, energy, and focus.
- **Aim for 30 plant-based foods per week:** This might sound like a lot, but remember, every herb, spice, fruit, veg, nut, seed, grain, and legume counts! Diversity feeds your gut microbiome, which plays a vital role in hormone metabolism, immune function, mental health, and inflammation levels. An easy way to hit your 30 is to think

about sprinkling in variety – for instance, add mixed seeds to porridge, herbs to dinner, or a handful of frozen veg into soups and sauces.

- **Pair movement with daily tasks:** You don't need a gym membership or hour-long blocks to move your body. Weave it into your day. Try doing counter push-ups while the kettle boils or dancing with the kids while making dinner. Short bursts of movement help release endorphins, protect joint mobility, and support circulation.

'I Don't Feel Like Myself Anymore': The Peri/Menopausal Years

Your kids are now older and life seems steadier on the surface, but you still feel wiped out or unable to find time for you – what's going on? This isn't just middle age. It's motherhood after the superhuman years, compounded by hormonal transitions and often decades of under-nourishment. The consequences matter and they can't and shouldn't be ignored.

I hear women say to me in clinic, 'I don't feel like me anymore' or 'I've lost all motivation.' Unfortunately, this is a common phenomenon and is the result of the slow fallout of long-term depletion combined with a sense of loss of purpose which is so entwined with your babies from the day they are born.

This stage is where it all converges and it's not easy. You are still supporting your children, but are now also navigating adolescence, possibly ageing parents, and career demands. There is less sleep urgency, but it has been replaced with subtle shifts in memory, mood, joints, and skin, and you find yourself in a body that feels weaker, achier, and slower to recover. The symptoms have come on so fast yet, at the same time, crept in so slowly. I hear you and I see you. It's OK – you have still got this and there's a lot you can do to recover, heal, and find yourself again.

For me, self-care isn't about spa days or candles (though I love those too); it's the small, consistent habits that keep me steady. My non-negotiables? Movement in some form every day – even if it's just a walk with my dog. I also make sure I get outside for fresh air daily, even if it's just 10 minutes – that bit of space and sky helps clear my head. I ensure I have a proper wind-down at night – no screens, just a book or some deep breaths – and time, even 10 minutes, to journal or sit in silence and check in with myself. These aren't luxuries. They're how I anchor myself – and I protect them fiercely now, because I've learnt the hard way what happens when I don't.

What the science says

There is a clinical cost of 'no time for me' by the stage of peri/menopause. As we saw in the previous chapter, after 40, women naturally lose some muscle mass each year and our joints may feel stiffer or achier as a result. This can also be due to long-standing poor posture habits or core weakness, not just ageing.

You might feel foggy, irritable, or forgetful – not because you are imagining it or 'losing it', but because your brain's chemical environment is adjusting to the hormonal fluctuations (revisit Chapter 6 for more on brain fog).

Oestrogen levels gently begin to fluctuate in your 40s and that can affect your energy, blood sugar, and fat distribution. Falling levels of oestrogen and progesterone can also disrupt your brain's ability to regulate sleep.

What many women don't realize is that cardiovascular disease is the leading cause of death in women over 50 and our risk increases sharply after menopause.[4] That's partly due to the natural drop in oestrogen, which previously helped protect our arteries. As levels fall, we become more vulnerable to high blood pressure, cholesterol build-up, strokes, and heart attacks. In fact, after menopause, our risk of heart disease catches up with men's – and, in some cases, overtakes it. The kicker? For decades, women were underrepresented in clinical trials on heart disease, which means our symptoms often go unrecognized, our risks underplayed, and our care delayed. This is why 'no time for me' has a clinical cost. Your heart health matters – and it's not selfish to protect it.

The good news is that your body is incredibly responsive to change, even in your 40s and 50s. You have not missed your window to reclaim yourself. You can absolutely feel better than you do now, more like yourself, and be the healthiest version of you even in the thick of the menopause years. With the right support, you can rebuild muscle mass, support brain clarity and mood, protect your bones, boost energy and focus, and prevent or reduce the risk of future health risks.

Eating to feel energized

You have cooked for everyone for years – now it's time to properly nourish you, not with diets or weight-loss jabs and pills, but with steady, hormone-friendly food that gives your body what it needs. The goal is balanced plates with more protein and fewer ultra-processed foods.

Nutrient	Why you need it now	Where to get it
Protein	Protects muscle, supports hormones	Eggs, yoghurt, tofu, beans, chicken, lentils
Calcium + vitamin D	Builds bones, supports nerves and mood	Dairy, fortified milks, greens, oily fish, sunshine
Fibre	Supports gut health, stabilizes mood and blood sugar	Wholegrains, veg, fruits, pulses
Omega-3s	Protects the brain and skin, supports mood	Oily fish, flaxseed, walnuts
Magnesium	Supports sleep, reduces anxiety and muscle tension	Dark chocolate, leafy greens, nuts

Daily movement

Remember, movement = energy, strength, and confidence, so try to incorporate daily exercise to really feel the benefits. A six-pack is not the goal here – it's about being able to move through life with ease and vitality.

So, how can you weave this into your day?

- **Take a 10-minute walk after meals:** This is great for blood sugar control.
- **Do bodyweight strength moves:** Exercises such as squats, lunges, or wall push-ups two to three times a week will really make a difference in building your strength.

- **Build in yoga or Pilates once a week:** As we age, balance naturally declines. Yoga or Pilates are powerful ways to support your muscles and joints in the long term and help with posture.
- **Have 'movement snacks' throughout the day:** Getting just a few minutes of movement in when you can – such as balancing on one leg when brushing your teeth or doing 10 squats while waiting for the kettle to boil – can really make a difference.

You don't need a gym or fancy equipment, you just need to start where you are, with what you have, and go from there.

What the science says

- **Strength training:** Supports your joints and protects your bones which are at risk during perimenopause and beyond. Even short bursts of resistance work can make a difference.[5]
- **Cardio exercise:** Keeps the heart and brain sharp, which suffer in this phase due to lower oestrogen levels.
- **Mobility:** Keeps you flexible and helps with pain management.

Protecting your sleep

Alongside falling levels of oestrogen and progesterone, there are several ways our sleep suffers in peri/menopause:

- Hot flushes and night sweats can jolt you awake during the night.
- Mood shifts, anxiety, and racing thoughts are common in perimenopause and can interfere with falling or staying asleep.

- Natural melatonin (which is the sleep hormone) production declines with age.
- Nocturia (waking to pee more than once a night) may increase due to changes in pelvic floor and bladder function.
- The mental load of life – work, caregiving, hormonal teens, ageing parents – impacts rest and recovery.

Thankfully, there are some simple things that can help to support your sleep at this stage:

- **Keep your bedroom cool, dark and calm:** A fan or cooling pillow can help with hot flushes.
- **Stick to a regular sleep–wake cycle:** Try to commit to this, even on weekends.
- **Avoid caffeine after 2pm and limit alcohol:** Both caffeine and alcohol disrupt deep sleep.
- **Build a wind-down routine:** Try reading, journaling, or gentle stretching instead of scrolling.
- **Take time to unload your thoughts:** Writing them down before bed can quiet a racing mind.
- **Try magnesium glycinate or calming herbs like ashwagandha (if appropriate):** These help to promote sleep and relaxation.
- **Eat foods that support sleep:** Bananas, oats, almonds, and pumpkin seeds are all good options.
- **Practise deep breathing or alternate nostril breathing:** This helps to calm your nervous system.
- **Consider cognitive behavioural therapy for insomnia (CBT-I):** This is a proven, effective treatment for sleep issues and available on the NHS in the UK.
- **Talk to your doctor about HRT or other support options:** If hormonal symptoms are disturbing your sleep, there are options available, so please do reach out.

In short, getting proper sleep, consistent movement, strength training, and eating a diet rich in fibre, protein, and omega-3s, can make a huge difference in this phase. Of course, if symptoms persist or worsen, check in with your doctor to rule out any underlying medical causes and to review whether there are medical or complementary interventions that could help.

What you can do

- **Keep it simple:** Small changes all add up – try adding in some chia seeds and nuts and berries to porridge, choosing wholegrain bread or pasta over white, adding protein to every meal, and drinking more water.
- **Take a 20-minute walk in daylight:** Light is medicine for your brain. Morning daylight resets your circadian rhythm, boosts serotonin, and improves sleep quality at night – which, in turn, sharpens focus and memory. Just 20 minutes outside before 10am makes a difference – you could even try standing on the doorstep with a cup of tea first thing.
- **Support collagen production naturally:** Collagen is an essential building block for good hair, nails, and skin. When oestrogen drops in the lead-up to menopause, collagen levels can fall too. Try to focus on the following to help your body make collagen:

  - protein from lean meat, fish, eggs, dairy, tofu, beans, or lentils
  - vitamin C found in berries, citrus fruits, broccoli, and peppers
  - zinc and copper, from nuts, seeds, wholegrains, and shellfish
  - iron and B12 (this is especially important if you're plant-based)
  - good hydration, which helps skin stay plump and elastic

I know that collagen supplements are popular, and some studies suggest that hydrolyzed collagen peptides may improve skin elasticity and hydration when taken consistently, but they're not a replacement for the basics and work best alongside good nutrition and rest. (If you're breastfeeding or on medication, check with your doctor before starting any new supplement.)

Punam's Prescription

Simplify your skincare routine

As I've said, all you really need is a gentle cleanser, a moisturizer, and a daily SPF. If possible, use products which contain ceramides, hyaluronic acid, and niacinamide:

- **Ceramides:** These are natural fats that sit in the outer layer of your skin. Think of them as the 'mortar' holding the skin 'bricks' together. They help keep the skin's barrier strong so moisture doesn't escape and irritants don't get in. When oestrogen drops, barrier function can weaken, and ceramides help replace what's lost.
- **Hyaluronic acid:** This helps your skin hold on to water. It acts like a sponge, drawing moisture into the skin and keeping it there. Hyaluronic acid helps skin feel more hydrated, softer, and smoother, and can make dryness and fine lines less noticeable. It doesn't create moisture on its own, but it helps your skin make better use of the moisture that's already there.
- **Niacinamide (a form of vitamin B3):** This helps strengthen the skin's barrier, support even tone, reduce redness, and improve texture. It also helps regulate oil production and can support skin immunity. It's a great all-rounder for stressed, sensitive, or ageing skin.

Together, these ingredients help address the common signs many women notice when hormones shift: dryness, dullness, sensitivity, and loss of elasticity.

If you want to choose products that contain ceramides, hyaluronic acid, and niacinamide, you might look for daily moisturizers or serums that combine them. These ingredients work well together: hyaluronic acid hydrates, ceramides lock that hydration in, and niacinamide supports barrier function and overall skin resilience. You can use these ingredients safely as part of your daily skincare routine. If you have very sensitive or reactive skin, start with a gentle formulation and introduce one product at a time to see how your skin responds.

Focus on micro-goals

When you're feeling low, overwhelmed, or just utterly depleted, the idea of doing something big for your health can feel impossible. That's where micro-goals come in. These are tiny, manageable actions that take just a few minutes but can create a ripple effect on your energy, mood, and motivation. You're not aiming for perfection here – you're just aiming to start.

Try these:

- **A brisk 2-minute walk:** Step outside or even pace around your house or garden. The movement will help reset your nervous system, get blood flowing, and give you a little lift.
- **A quick stretch:** Reach up to the ceiling, roll your shoulders back, or do a gentle forward fold. This helps release physical tension and brings you back into your body.
- **No skipping meals:** Even if it's a small handful of nuts and a banana, your brain and body need fuel to function. Try to eat something within one to two hours of waking, and don't go long stretches without food – it only adds to the fog and fatigue.
- **Hydrate:** Start the day with a glass of room-temperature water before your tea or coffee. Dehydration is a silent drain on energy, skin, and focus.
- **One nourishing decision:** This could be stepping away

from your phone at bedtime, taking your supplements, or opening the window for some fresh air. It doesn't have to be huge to be helpful.

These small, low-pressure steps aren't just a bridge back to your health – they *are* your health. Think of them as daily acts of self-respect. When done consistently, they add up and you'll start to feel the difference.

Eat mindfully

Let's be honest – most mums don't 'eat meals' so much as inhale whatever's closest. This is survival eating. But the problem is, when eating becomes a background task – something done on the go, standing at the sink, or while wiping a toddler's face – it stops nourishing you properly.

Mindful eating isn't just about being fancy or zen. It's about giving your body the chance to rest, digest, and absorb. Your digestive system only works well when your body feels safe and calm – not rushed or on high alert. When you sit down, take a breath and chew slowly. You're not just feeding your body – you're giving your nervous system a break. This is something I talk to patients about all the time, and I've learnt to remind myself too: you are allowed to eat a proper meal, sitting down at the table, with both hands free.

Here's how to reclaim mealtimes:

- **Eat at the table, even if it's just once a day:** Sitting down sends a powerful signal to your body: I matter. This matters.
- **Share meals with your kids when you can:** Not only is it good for their development and eating habits, it's a reminder that you're not just the feeder. You're allowed to eat too.
- **Chew slowly:** Digestion starts in your mouth. When we rush, we swallow air, overload our gut, and miss the satiety signals that tell us we've had enough.

- **Put your phone down:** Screens distract your brain from the experience of eating, which can make you feel less full and more frazzled.
- **Make food feel like care, not a chore:** Play music, light a candle, or use your favourite mug. Small rituals can make even a thrown-together lunch feel more like a moment for you.

Eating slowly, regularly, and mindfully can help reduce bloating, improve gut health, balance blood sugar, and, just as importantly, remind you that your needs matter.

Because when you treat your mealtimes with respect, you start treating yourself with respect too.

Final Thoughts

When it comes to self-care and carving out time for yourself, you don't need to overhaul your life. You don't need a spa retreat or a 12-week paid plan. You just need a moment, a meal, a walk, a deep breath, and a yes, to yourself. Across all stages, from postnatal recovery to the menopause years:

- Nourishing your body with protein, healthy fats, fibre, and micronutrients supports mood, energy, hormone balance, and repair.
- Daily movement, especially through strength and mobility work, protects against pain, frailty, metabolic issues, and bone loss.
- Giving space for your mind – through sleep, sunlight, or breathwork – can change your entire nervous system response.

Your health is foundational. It doesn't need perfection, it needs attention and small acts of consistent care. As you have done and still do for those you love, do it for you too.

Final Note

As we come to the end of this book, I want to return to where we began. Maternal health does not begin and end with pregnancy or the first year after birth. It stretches across every season of motherhood, because we grow and change alongside our children. Our bodies, minds, and identities are constantly adapting, but the support we receive rarely keeps pace. Motherhood was never meant to be a solo load, and yet so many women are carrying it alone. That is the motherhood health penalty.

We can't keep putting the burden of resilience solely on mothers. If we truly want to support families, we need to treat maternal well-being as a foundation of public health, not a personal luxury. Imagine what the world might look like if postnatal care extended beyond a single six-week check. If women had routine access to pelvic health physios, mental health checks, and breastfeeding support. If communities and systems were designed to reduce isolation – from drop-in centres to safe, welcoming spaces for mums to connect without pressure. If we divided labour at home and at work, so that raising children wasn't something women do on top of everything else, in the cracks of their own lives. If peri/menopause was recognized early and supported properly, rather than brushed off. If maternal health was treated not as a niche issue, but as a cornerstone of public health. If you're a policymaker, employer, educator, or health leader reading this: mothers deserve more, and at every season of their mothering life. Healthier mums build healthier families – and that benefits everyone.

Here is what I want you to take away from this book, from a mum who has been there and from a GP who has sat with thousands of women who thought they were the only ones struggling: you are doing something extraordinary – loving, holding, guiding, raising, worrying, juggling, and growing. You are doing enough. You are more than enough and you are never as alone as you might sometimes feel.

Motherhood is full of contradictions: overwhelming love alongside overwhelming loneliness, deep connection alongside deep exhaustion, joy woven tightly with fear, pain, guilt, and doubt. But, among it all, try to remember who you are beyond motherhood. You are a whole person. A woman with a history, loves, talents, dreams, humour, quirks, and needs.

Motherhood is a chapter of your life – a beautiful one – but it's not the entirety of you. Reconnecting with the parts of yourself that feel lost is not indulgent. It's necessary. And it's powerful. Because when your children see you valuing your health, your joy, and your sense of self, it gives them permission to do the same.

While I was writing this book, my own journey took an unexpected turn. I was diagnosed with breast cancer. Suddenly, alongside being a GP, a writer, and a mother, I was also a patient – navigating treatment, fear, uncertainty, and recovery. What struck me most was how, even in the midst of serious illness, motherhood doesn't pause. You still show up. You still pack lunches, offer reassurance, and hold emotions that aren't just your own. When you have young children, you don't always get the luxury of falling apart – even when your body and heart are asking for rest. That experience deepened everything I wanted to say in these pages.

If you are a mother reading this while carrying illness, grief, exhaustion, mental load, or simply too much, I see you. I am holding space for you. Everything in this book is grounded in what I practise, what I believe in, and what has helped me and the women I care for. I have written it with honesty, compassion, and love – from one mum to another.

Motherhood is a journey of ups and downs, grief and joy, loss and becoming. It is demanding, beautiful, stretching, and transformative. You are not meant to do it perfectly. You are not meant to do it alone. And you are allowed to need care, support, and understanding – at every stage.

I hope this book has helped you feel seen, supported, and a little less alone. I hope it's reminded you that you're not imagining things and you don't have to keep struggling in silence. There is help. There is healing. And there is still so much of you here, waiting to be reclaimed.

We are in this together.

Punam xx

Acknowledgements

First and foremost, I want to thank my children, Aarish and Ellora, for making me a mother. You are my greatest teachers and my deepest source of inspiration. I have grown alongside you both, and everything I know about love, patience, humility, and resilience has been shaped by being your mum. Thank you for your understanding, your hugs, and for giving me pockets of space to write when I needed them. This book exists because you allowed me to experience the beautiful journey of motherhood – a journey that has allowed me to connect with other mums, all growing together.

To my husband Sandesh, thank you for sharing the load with me and for being my constant support through every season. Thank you for backing my ideas, believing in my vision, and holding things steady at home while I chased words, deadlines, and dreams. I could not have written this book without you.

To my mum – my greatest inspiration and my closest friend – thank you for continuing to guide me as I grow. Your wisdom, strength, and love have shaped me in more ways than I can ever express. If I can be even half the mum you have been to us, I'll be winning.

To my dad, thank you for your quiet strength, your steadiness, and the values you instilled in me long before I became a mother myself. Your work ethic, integrity, and calm presence have shaped who I am more than you probably realize, and I carry that into my parenting every day.

To my sister, Preeti, thank you for being my go-to for childcare and for always stepping in, often at the last minute, to give me the space I needed to write this book. Your support, patience, and willingness to review it along the way have meant more than you know. You're the best massi in the world.

To my friends, and especially my mum friends, thank you for reminding me time and again that we are not meant to do this alone. For the honesty, the laughter, the voice notes, the shared tears, and the constant reassurance that we are all making it up as we go along.

To my best friend, my ride-or-die, George, thank you for always being there in every way that matters. For listening without judgement, swapping mum rants, holding space on the days when it all felt like too much, and for reviewing this book at every stage with such care and honesty. Doing motherhood alongside you has made it lighter.

To my agent and the team at BBM – what a ride. I couldn't have done this without you.

To my wonderful team at DK, thank you for believing in me and for backing this book so wholeheartedly. And a special, heartfelt thank you to my editor, Julia Kellaway; a fellow mum who truly got it. You guided me with care, kept me grounded, and made the process not just manageable, but genuinely enjoyable. I couldn't have asked for a better person to walk this journey with.

This book was written with love, lived experience, and deep respect for mothers everywhere. Thank you to everyone who held me up while I wrote it.

References

Introduction

1. 'More than a third of women experience lasting health problems after childbirth, new research shows', World Health Organization, 7 December 2023, available at: www.who.int/news/item/07-12-2023-more-than-a-third-of-women-experience-lasting-health-problems-after-childbirth
   Devi Sridhar, 'Why does postnatal care only last a few weeks? New data shows it should be years', *The Guardian*, 24 May 2024, available at: www.theguardian.com/commentisfree/article/2024/may/24/postnatal-care-weeks-data-years-health-women-nhs.

Chapter 1: 'I Had a Difficult Birth'

1. Cheryl Tatano Beck, Sue Watson, and Robert K. Gable, 'Traumatic childbirth and its aftermath: Is there anything positive?', *The Journal of Perinatal Education*, June 2018, 27(3), pp. 175–84, available at: pmc.ncbi.nlm.nih.gov/articles/PMC6193358/.
2. Helen Stanley, 'What is a birth debrief – and why might I need one?', Birth Trauma Association, n.d., available at: birthtraumaassociation.org/news-campaigns/birth-trauma-inquiry-akt3f.
3. All-Party Parliamentary Group on Birth Trauma, 'Listen to mums: Ending the postcode lottery on perinatal care', 13 May 2024, available at: www.theo-clarke.org.uk/birth-trauma-report.
4. 'The management of third- and fourth-degree perineal tears: Green-top guideline no. 29', Royal College of Obstetricians & Gynaecologists, June 2015, available at: www.rcog.org.uk/media/5jeb5hzu/gtg-29.pdf.
   Vasanth Andrews, Abdul H. Sultan, Ranee Thakar, et al., 'Occult anal sphincter injuries – myth or reality?', *BJOG*, February 2006, 113(2), pp. 195–200, available at: pubmed.ncbi.nlm.nih.gov/16411998/.
5. 'Left unchecked – why maternal mental health matters', Healthwatch England, March 2023, available at: nds.healthwatch.co.uk/sites/default/files/reports_library/20230315%20Left%20unchecked%20briefing.pdf.
6. Matthew Limb, 'Maternity care "fell short of expectations", regulator's annual survey finds', *BMJ*, 28 November 2024, 387, q2680, available at: www.bmj.com/content/387/bmj.q2680;
   All-Party Parliamentary Group on Birth Trauma, 'Listen to mums: Ending the postcode lottery on perinatal care', 13 May 2024, available at: www.theo-clarke.org.uk/files/2024-05/Birth%20Trauma%20Inquiry%20Report%20for%20Publication_May13_2024.pdf.

Chapter 2: 'I'm Tired All the Time'

1. Elizabeth C. Meyer, 'Depleted mother syndrome: What it is & how to cope', ChoosingTherapy.com, 29 July 2024, available at: www.choosingtherapy.com/depleted-mother-syndrome/#:~:text=You%20might%20have%20depleted%20mother,just%20too%20much%20for%20you;
'Mom burnout & substance abuse: What you need to know', Caron, n.d., available at: www.caron.org/addiction-101/substance-abuse/mom-burnout-substance-abuse-what-you-need-to-know#:~:text=Mom%20burnout%20sometimes%20called%20depleted,resources%20for%20coping%20with%20it.

2. Jodi A. Mindell, Avi Sadeh, Robert Kwon, et al., 'Cross-cultural comparison of maternal sleep', *Sleep*, 1 November 2013, 36(11), pp. 1699–706, available at: pmc.ncbi.nlm.nih.gov/articles/PMC3792388/#:~:text=%2C%20P%20%3E%200.05.-,Sleep%20Disturbances,lack%20of%20enthusiasm%20(5.5%25).

3. 'Mothers bear the brunt of the "mental load", managing 7 in 10 household tasks', University of Bath, 12 December 2024, available at: www.bath.ac.uk/announcements/mothers-bear-the-brunt-of-the-mental-load-managing-7-in-10-household-tasks/#:~:text=Key%20Findings,%2C%20who%20manage%20just%2045%25;
Ana Catalano Weeks and Leah Ruppanner, 'A typology of US parents' mental loads: Core and episodic cognitive labor', *Journal of Marriage and Family*, 12 December 2024, 87(3),
pp. 966–89, available at: onlinelibrary.wiley.com/doi/10.1111/jomf.13057.

4. R. F. Baumeister, E. Bratslavsky, M. Muraven, et al., 'Ego depletion: Is the active self a limited resource?', *Journal of Personality and Social Psychology*, 1998, 74(5), pp. 1252–65, available at pubmed.ncbi.nlm.nih.gov/9599441/.

5. Yee Mellor, 'Perimenopause: Symptoms and management', *The Pharmaceutical Journal*, 24 January 2023, 310(7969), available at: pharmaceutical-journal.com/article/ld/perimenopause-symptoms-and-management.

6. Bryan Robinson, 'Why neuroscientists say, "Boredom Is good for your brain's health"', *Forbes*, 2 September 2020, available at: www.forbes.com/sites/bryanrobinson/2020/09/02/why-neuroscientists-say-boredom-is-good-for-your-brains-health/.

7. R. I. M. Dunbar, 'Breaking bread: The functions of social eating', *Adaptive Human Behavior and Physiology*, 11 March 2017, 3(3), pp. 198–211, available at: pmc.ncbi.nlm.nih.gov/articles/PMC6979515/;
Kimberly A. Dill-McFarland, Zheng-Zheng Tang, Julia H. Kemis, et al. 'Close social relationships correlate with human gut microbiota composition', *Scientific Reports*, 24 January 2019, 9(703), available at: www.nature.com/articles/s41598-018-37298-9.

Chapter 3: 'Nothing Looks or Feels Normal Down There'

1. 'RCOG calling for action to reduce number of women living with poor pelvic floor health', Royal College of Obstetricians & Gynaecologists, 2 February 2023, available at: www.rcog.org.uk/news/rcog-calling-for-action-to-reduce-number-of-women-living-with-poor-pelvic-floor-health/.

2. 'Perineal tears during childbirth', Royal College of Obstetricians & Gynaecologists, n.d., available at: www.rcog.org.uk/for-the-public/perineal-tears-and-episiotomies-in-childbirth/perineal-tears-during-childbirth.

3. David H. Thom and Guri Rortveit, 'Prevalence of postpartum urinary incontinence: A systematic review', *Acta Obstetricia et Gynecologica Scandinavica*, December 2010, 89(12), pp. 1511–22, available at: pubmed.ncbi.nlm.nih.gov/21050146;
S. Brown, D. Gartland, S. Perlen, et al., 'Consultation about urinary and faecal incontinence in the year after childbirth: A cohort study', *BJOG*, June 2015, 122(7), pp. 954–62, available at: pubmed.ncbi.nlm.nih.gov/25039427.

4. 'Body after birth: Incontinence, vagina, and more', NCT, n.d., available at: www.nct.org.uk/information/pregnancy/body-pregnancy/10-truths-leaking-urine-pregnancy-and-after-birth#:~:text=5.-,Urinary%20incontinence%20is%20super%20common,and%20almost%20half%20with%20friends%20.

5. Donelle Cross, Nasreena Waheed, Michelle Krake, et al., 'Effectiveness of supervised Kegel exercises using bio-feedback versus unsupervised Kegel exercises on stress urinary incontinence: A quasi-experimental study', *International Urogynecology Journal*, 8 July 2022, 34(4), pp. 913–20, available at: pmc.ncbi.nlm.nih.gov/articles/PMC9266083/#:~:text=Evidence%20suggests%20that%20Kegel%20exercises,floor%20exercise%20programme%20%5B12%5D.

6. Louise Carroll, Cliona O'Sullivan, Catherine Doody, et al., 'Pelvic organ prolapse: The lived experience', *PloS One*, 2 November 2022, 17(11), available at: pmc.ncbi.nlm.nih.gov/articles/PMC9629641.

7. 'Facts and Figures', Breast Cancer UK, n.d., available at: www.breastcanceruk.org.uk/about-breast-cancer/facts-figures-and-qas/facts-and-figures/#:~:text=Global%20breast%20cancer%20statistics,deaths%20among%20women%20(1).

Chapter 4: 'I'll Never Have Sex Again ... Or Will I?'

1. Mojdeh Banaei, Nourossadat Kariman, Giti Ozgoli, et al., 'Prevalence of postpartum dyspareunia: A systematic review and meta-analysis', *International Journal of Gynaecology and Obstetrics*, April 2021, 153(1), pp. 14–24, available at: pubmed.ncbi.nlm.nih.gov/33300122.

2. Nada Saleh Albalawi, Maram Ati Almohammadi, and Ahmad Raja Albalawi, 'Comparison of the efficacy of vaginal hyaluronic acid to estrogen for the treatment of vaginal atrophy in postmenopausal women: A systematic review', *Cureus*, 27 August 2023, 15(8), available at: www.ncbi.nlm.nih.gov/pmc/articles/PMC10520994/;

Ayane Cristine Alves Sarmento, Márcia Farina Kamilos, Ana Paula Ferreira Costa, et al., 'Use of moisturizers and lubricants for vulvovaginal atrophy', *Frontiers in Reproductive Health*, 23 December 2021, 3, 781353, available at: www.ncbi.nlm.nih.gov/pmc/articles/PMC9580673/;

Liisa Lehtoranta, Reeta Ala-Jaakkola, Arja Laitila, et al., 'Healthy vaginal microbiota and influence of probiotics across the female life span', *Frontiers in Microbiology*, 8 April 2022, 13, available at: www.frontiersin.org/articles/10.3389/fmicb.2022.819958/full;

Peng Liu, Yune Lu, Rongguo Li, et al., 'Use of probiotic lactobacilli in the treatment of vaginal infections: *In vitro* and *in vivo* investigations', *Frontiers in Cellular and Infection Microbiology*, 3 April 2023, 13, available at: www.frontiersin.org/articles/10.3389/fcimb.2023.1153894/full;

Zhaojun Mei and Dandan Li, 'The role of probiotics in vaginal health', *Frontiers in Cellular and Infection Microbiology*, 28 July 2022, 12, 963868, available at: www.ncbi.nlm.nih.gov/pmc/articles/PMC9366906/.

3. Emily Nagoski, *Come as You Are: The bestselling guide to the new science that will transform your sex life* (London: Scribe UK, 2015).

Chapter 5: 'Everything Hurts'

1. Jorun Bakken Sperstad, Merete Kolberg Tennfjord, Gunvor Hilde, et al., 'Diastasis recti abdominis during pregnancy and 12 months after childbirth: Prevalence, risk factors and report of lumbopelvic pain', *British Journal of Sports Medicine*, 20 June 2016, 50(17), pp. 1092–96, available at: pmc.ncbi.nlm.nih.gov/articles/PMC5013086/.

2. P. Katonis, A. Kampouroglou, A. Aggelopoulos, et al., 'Pregnancy-related low back pain', *Hippokratia*, July–September 2011, 15(3), pp. 205–10, available at: pmc.ncbi.nlm.nih.gov/articles/PMC3306025/.

3. Sarah Leyland, 'What's the menopause got to do with bone health?', Royal Osteoporosis Society, 22 March 2021, available at: theros.org.uk/blog/2021-03-22-what-s-the-menopause-got-to-do-with-bone-health/.

4. M. Julie Thornton, 'Estrogens and aging skin', *Dermato-endocrinology*, 1 April 2013, 5(2), pp. 264–70, available at: pmc.ncbi.nlm.nih.gov/articles/PMC3772914/.

5. M. S. LeBoff, S. L. Greenspan, K. L. Insogna, et al., 'The clinician's guide to prevention and treatment of osteoporosis', *Osteoporosis International*, 28 April 2022, 33(10), pp. 2049–102, available at: pmc.ncbi.nlm.nih.gov/articles/PMC9546973/.

6. 'Menopause: Identification and management', NICE, 12 November 2015, available at: www.nice.org.uk/guidance/ng23/chapter/recommendations.

Chapter 6: 'I'm Having Difficulty Concentrating'

1. Kristine Yaffe, Cherie M. Falvey, and Tina Hoang, 'Connections between sleep and cognition in older adults', *The Lancet Neurology*, October 2014, 13(10), pp. 1017–28, available at: www.thelancet.com/journals/laneur/article/PIIS1474-4422(14)70172-3/abstract.

2. Elseline Hoekzema, Erika Barba-Müller, Cristina Pozzobon, et al., 'Pregnancy leads to long-lasting changes in human brain structure', *Nature Neuroscience*, February 2017, 20(2), pp. 287–96, available at: pubmed.ncbi.nlm.nih.gov/27991897/.

3. A. M. Williamson and Anne-Marie Feyer, 'Moderate sleep deprivation produces impairments in cognitive and motor performance equivalent to legally prescribed levels of alcohol intoxication', *Occupational and Environmental Medicine*, 2000, 57, pp. 649–55, available at: pmc.ncbi.nlm.nih.gov/articles/instance/1739867/pdf/v057p00649.pdf.

4. Sasha J. Davies, Jarrad Ag Lum, Helen Skouteris, et al., 'Cognitive impairment during pregnancy: A meta-analysis', *The Medical Journal of Australia*, 15 January 2018, 208(1), pp. 35–40, available at: pubmed.ncbi.nlm.nih.gov/29320671/.

5. Alison Andrew, Sarah Cattan, Monica Costa Dias, et al., 'Parents, especially mothers, paying heavy price for lockdown', IFS, 27 May 2020, available at: ifs.org.uk/news/parents-especially-mothers-paying-heavy-price-lockdown.

6. Nelson Cowan, 'The magical mystery four: How is working memory capacity limited, and why?', *Current Directions in Psychological Science*, 1 February 2010, 19(1), pp. 51–7, available at: pmc.ncbi.nlm.nih.gov/articles/PMC2864034.

7. Gail A. Greendale, Richard G. Wight, Mei-Hua Huang, et al., 'Menopause-associated symptoms and cognitive performance: Results from the study of women's health across the nation', *American Journal of Epidemiology*, 1 June 2010, 171(11), pp. 1214–24, available at: pubmed.ncbi.nlm.nih.gov/20442205/.

8. Miriam T. Weber, Pauline M. Maki, and Michael P. McDermott, 'Cognition and mood in perimenopause: A systematic review and meta-analysis', *The Journal of Steroid Biochemistry and Molecular Biology*, 14 June 2013, 142, pp. 90–8, available at: pmc.ncbi.nlm.nih.gov/articles/PMC3830624/.

9. Lianlian Lei, Amanda N. Leggett, and Donovan T. Maust, 'A national profile of sandwich generation caregivers providing care to both older adults and children', *Journal of the American Geriatrics Society*, 25 November 2022, 71(3), pp. 799–809, available at: pmc.ncbi.nlm.nih.gov/articles/PMC10023280/.

10. Stephen Monsell, 'Task switching', *Trends in Cognitive Sciences*, March 2003, 7(3), pp. 134–40, available at: pubmed.ncbi.nlm.nih.gov/12639695/.

11. 'Menopause: Identification and management', NICE, 12 November 2015, available at: www.nice.org.uk/guidance/ng23/.

Chapter 7: 'I'm Feeling Scared'

1. 'Baby blues and postpartum depression: Mood disorders and pregnancy', Johns Hopkins Medicine, 2026, available at: https://www.hopkinsmedicine. org/health/wellness-and-prevention/postpartum-mood-disorders-what-new-moms-need-to-know?

2. Shefaly Shorey, Cornelia Yin Ing Chee, Esperanza Debby Ng, et al., 'Prevalence and incidence of postpartum depression among healthy mothers: A systematic review and meta-analysis', *Journal of Psychiatric Research*, September 2018, 104, pp. 235–48, available at: www.sciencedirect.com/science/article/abs/pii/S0022395618304928?via%3Dihub.

3. Fanie Collardeau, Bryony Corbyn, John Abramowitz, et al., 'Maternal unwanted and intrusive thoughts of infant-related harm, obsessive-compulsive disorder and depression in the perinatal period: Study protocol', *BMC Psychiatry*, 21 March 2019, 19(1), p. 94, available at: pmc.ncbi.nlm.nih.gov/articles/PMC6429780/.

4. Elseline Hoekzema, Erika Barba-Müller, Cristina Pozzobon, et al., 'Pregnancy leads to long-lasting changes in human brain structure', *Nature Neuroscience*, 19 December 2016, 20, pp. 287–96.

5. Joyce T. Bromberger, Howard M. Kravitz, Yue-Fang Chang, et al., 'Major depression during and after the menopausal transition: Study of Women's Health Across the Nation (SWAN)', *Psychological Medicine*, 9 February 2011, 41(9), pp. 1879–88, available at: pmc.ncbi.nlm.nih.gov/articles/PMC3584692/;
Ellen W. Freeman, 'Depression in the menopause transition: Risks in the changing hormone milieu as observed in the general population', *Women's Midlife Health*, 11 August 2015, 1, p. 2, available at: pmc.ncbi.nlm.nih.gov/articles/PMC6214217;
Yasmeen Badawy, Aimee Spector, Zishi Li, et al., 'The risk of depression in the menopausal stages: A systematic review and meta-analysis' *Journal of Affective Disorders*, July 2024, 357, pp. 126–33, available at: pubmed.ncbi.nlm.nih.gov/38642901/;
Lisa M. Shitomi-Jones, Clare Dolman, Ian Jones, et al., 'Exploration of first onsets of mania, schizophrenia spectrum disorders and major depressive disorder in perimenopause', *Nature Mental Health*, 15 August 2024, 2, pp. 1161–8, available at: www.nature.com/articles/s44220-024-00292-4 .

6. Terese Glatz and Melissa A. Lippold, 'Is more information always better? Associations among parents' online information searching, information overload, and self-efficacy', *International Journal of Behavioral Development*, 2023, 47(5), pp. 444–53, available at: journals.sagepub.com/doi/pdf/10.1177/01650254231190883;
Beatrice Beebe, Miriam Steele, Joseph Jaffe, et al., 'Maternal anxiety symptoms and mother-infant self- and interactive contingency', *Infant Mental Health Journal*, 8 March 2011, 32(2), pp. 174–206, available at: pmc.ncbi.nlm.nih.gov/articles/PMC4431701/ (accessed January 2026); Steven F. Warren and Nancy C.

Brady, 'The role of maternal responsivity in the development of children with intellectual disabilities', *Mental Retardation and Developmental Disabilities Research Reviews*, 2007, 13(4), pp. 330–8, available at: pmc.ncbi.nlm.nih.gov/articles/PMC7382819/.

7. Office of the Surgeon General, 'The current state of parental stress & well-being', in: *Parents Under Pressure: The US Surgeon General's advisory on the mental health & well-being of parents* (Washington, DC, US Department of Health and Human Services, 2024).

Chapter 8: 'I Feel Like I'm "Always On"'

1. Erika Barba-Müller, Sinéad Craddock, Susanna Carmona, et al., 'Brain plasticity in pregnancy and the postpartum period: Links to maternal caregiving and mental health', *Archives of Women's Mental Health*, 14 July 2018, 22(2), pp. 289–99, available at: pmc.ncbi.nlm.nih.gov/articles/PMC6440938/; Elseline Hoekzema, Erika Barba-Müller, Cristina Pozzobon, et al., 'Pregnancy leads to long-lasting changes in human brain structure', *Nature Neuroscience*, February 2017, 20(2), pp. 287–96, available at: pubmed.ncbi.nlm.nih.gov/27991897/.

2. Katharine Ann James, Juliet Ilena Stromin, Nina Steenkamp, et al., 'Understanding the relationships between physiological and psychosocial stress, cortisol and cognition', *Frontiers in Endocrinology*, 6 March 2023, 14, 1085950, available at: pmc.ncbi.nlm.nih.gov/articles/PMC10025564/.

3. Megan Clapp, Nadia Aurora, Lindsey Herrera, et al., 'Gut microbiota's effect on mental health: The gut-brain axis', *Clinics and Practice*, 15 September 2017, 7(4), p. 987, available at: pmc.ncbi.nlm.nih.gov/articles/PMC5641835/.

4. Daniel J. Siegel, *The Developing Mind: How relationships and the brain interact to shape who we are* (New York, The Guilford Press, 2012).

5. Bessel Van der Kolk, *The Body Keeps the Score: Brain, mind, and body in the healing of trauma* (New York, Penguin Group USA, 2015).

6. Isabelle Roskam, Joyce Aguiar, Ege Akgun, et al., 'Parental burnout around the globe: A 42-country study', *Affective Science*, 18 March 2021, 2, pp. 58–79, available at: link.springer.com/article/10.1007/s42761-020-00028-4; Kate Sustersic Gawlik, Bernadette Mazurek Melnyk, and Alai Tan, 'Burnout and mental health in working parents: Risk factors and practice implications', *Journal of Pediatric Health Care*, January–February 2025, 39(1), pp. 41–50, available at: www.sciencedirect.com/science/article/pii/S0891524524001883; Agata Maria Urbanowicz, Rebecca Shankland, Jaynie Rance, et al., 'Cognitive behavioral stress management for parents: Prevention and reduction of parental burnout', *International Journal of Clinical and Health Psychology*, October–December 2023, 23(4), 100365, available at: www.sciencedirect.com/science/article/pii/S1697260023000017.

7. Petruța P. Rusu, Octav-Sorin Candel, Ionela Bogdan, et al., 'Parental stress and well-being: A meta-analysis', *Clinical Child and Family Psychology Review*, 8 March 2025, 28(2), pp. 255–74, available at: pmc.ncbi.nlm.nih.gov/articles/PMC12162691/.

8. D. W. Winnicott, 'The theory of the parent-infant relationship', *International Journal of Psycho Analysis*, 1960, 411, pp. 585–95, available at: tcf-website-media-library.s3.eu-west-2.amazonaws.com/wp-content/uploads/2021/09/21095241/; Winnicott-D.-1960.-The-Theory-of-the-Parent-Infant-Relationship.-International-Journal-of-Psycho-Analysis.-411.-pp.585-595-1.pdf.

Chapter 9: 'I Feel Isolated'

1. 'Invisible mothers: The state of invisibility', October 2023, Peanut, available at: storage.googleapis.com/peanut-assets/reports/UK%20-%20The%20State%20of%20Invisibility.pdf.
2. Chong Chen, Yasuhiro Mochizuki, Sumiyo Okawa, et al., 'Postpartum loneliness predicts future depressive symptoms: A nationwide Japanese longitudinal study', *Archives of Women's Mental Health*, June 2024, 27(3), pp. 447–57, available at: pubmed.ncbi.nlm.nih.gov/38279068/; Billie Lever Taylor, Louise M. Howard, Katherine Jackson, et al., 'Mums alone: Exploring the role of isolation and loneliness in the narratives of women diagnosed with perinatal depression', *Journal of Clinical Medicine*, 24 May 2021, 10(11), 2271, available at: pmc.ncbi.nlm.nih.gov/articles/PMC8197355/ (accessed January 2026); Ruth Naughton-Doe, Rebecca Nowland, Jacqueline Kent-Marvick, et al., 'Exploring perinatal loneliness as a key social determinant of perinatal mental ill health in the UK: Findings from a multidisciplinary consensus statement exercise that mapped knowledge about measurement, prevalence, antecedents, impacts and interventions, and agreed future priorities for research, policy and practice', *BMJ Open*, 2025, 15, 085669, available at: bmjopen.bmj.com/content/bmjopen/15/5/e085669.full.pdf.
3. Tiffany De Sousa Machado, Anna Chur-Hansen, and Clemence Due, 'First-time mothers' perceptions of social support: Recommendations for best practice', *Health Psychology Open*, 7 February 2020, 7(1), available at: pmc.ncbi.nlm.nih. gov/articles/PMC7008558/; Mehreen Zaigham, Karolina Linden, Helen Elden, et al., 'Trends in the quality of maternal and neonatal care in Sweden and Norway as compared to 12 WHO European countries: A cross-sectional survey investigating maternal perspectives during the COVID-19 pandemic', *Acta Obstetricia et Gynecologica Scandinavica*, December 2024, 103(12), pp. 2485–98, available at: pubmed. ncbi.nlm.nih.gov/39431577/; Anna Horakova, Hana Nemcova, Kristyna Hrdlickova, et al., 'State of perinatal mental health care in the WHO region of Europe: A scoping review', *Frontiers in Psychiatry*, 13 March 2024, 15, p. 1350036, available at: pubmed.ncbi.nlm. nih.gov/38544852/.
4. Leah D. Doane and Emma K. Adam, 'Loneliness and cortisol: Momentary, day-to-day, and trait associations', *Psychoneuroendocrinology*, 9 September

2009, 35(3), pp. 430–41, available at: pmc.ncbi.nlm.nih.gov/articles/PMC2841363/.

5. Suniya S. Luthar and Lucia Ciciolla, 'What it feels like to be a mother: Variations by children's developmental stages', *Developmental Psychology*, 2016, 52(1), pp. 143–54, available at: psycnet.apa.org/doiLanding?doi=10.1037%2Fdev0000062.

6. 'Mothers bear the brunt of the "mental load", managing 7 in 10 household tasks', University of Bath, 12 December 2024, available at: www.bath.ac.uk/announcements/mothers-bear-the-brunt-of-the-mental-load-managing-7-in-10-household-tasks/#:~:text=Key%20Findings,%2C%20who%20manage%20just%2045%25.

7. 'Men enjoy five hours more leisure time per week than women', Office for National Statistics, 9 January 2018, available at: www.ons.gov.uk/peoplepopulationandcommunity/wellbeing/articles/menenjoyfivehoursmoreleisuretimeperweekthanwomen/2018-01-09#:~:text=Though%20people%20living%20with%20children,child%20in%20their%20household%20was.

8. 'Shocking extent of loneliness faced by young mothers revealed', Co-operative Group Limited, 2 May 20218, available at: https://www.co-operative.coop/media/news-releases/shocking-extent-of-loneliness-faced-by-young-mothers-revealed

Chapter 10: 'There's No Time for Me'

1. Petruța P. Rusu, Octav-Sorin Candel, Ionela Bogdan, et al., 'Parental stress and well-being: A meta-analysis', *Clinical Child and Family Psychology Review*, 8 March 2025, 28(2), pp. 255–74, available at: pmc.ncbi.nlm.nih.gov/articles/PMC12162691/.

2. 'Pelvic floor dysfunction: Prevention and non-surgical management', NICE, 9 December 2021, available at: www.nice.org.uk/guidance/ng210.

3. Jiongxing Fu, Yan Zheng, Ying Gao, et al., 'Dietary fiber intake and gut microbiota in human health', *Microorganisms*, 18 December 2022, 10(12), 2507, available at: pmc.ncbi.nlm.nih.gov/articles/PMC9787832/.

4. 'Menopause and your heart', British Heart Foundation, 1 October 2023, available at: https://www.bhf.org.uk/informationsupport/support/women-with-a-heart-condition/menopause-and-heart-disease?

5. Erika Svensen, Christopher P. Koscien, Nima Alamdari, et al., 'A novel low-impact resistance exercise program increases strength and balance in females irrespective of menopause status', *Medicine & Science in Sports & Exercise*, March 2025, 57(3), pp. 501–13, available at: journals.lww.com/acsm-msse/fulltext/2025/03000/a_novel_low_impact_resistance_exercise_program.6.aspx;
Ana María Capel-Alcaraz, Héctor García-López, Adelaida María Castro-Sánchez, et al., 'The efficacy of strength exercises for reducing the symptoms of menopause: A systematic review', *Journal of Clinical Medicine*, 9 January 2023, 12(2), p. 548, available at: pmc.ncbi.nlm.nih.gov/articles/PMC9864448/.

Index